CARTILAGE REPA

CURRENT CONCEPTS

DJO PUBLICATIONS

A DJO Global, Inc. initiative
International Headquarters - London

www.DJOpublications.com

Project Manager: Francine Van Steenkiste
Book and Cover Design: Lee Millington / Gemma Hatherley
Illustrations: Gemma Hatherley
Production: Gemma Hatherley
Compositor: DJO Publications (DJO Global, Inc.)

First edition 2010

ISBN number: 978-0-9558873-1-4

Published by DJO Publications
1a Guildford Business Park
Guildford
Surrey
GU2 8XG
UK
www.DJOglobal.eu

Printed in the UK

CARTILAGE REPAIR

CURRENT CONCEPTS

EDITORS:

Mats Brittberg
MD, Professor
Cartilage Research Unit
Orthopaedic Department
Gothenburg University
Kungsbacka, Sweden

Andreas Imhoff
MD, Professor
Dept. of Orthopaedic Sports Medicine
Klinikum Rechts der Isar
University of Munich
Munich, Germany

Henning Madry
MD, Professor
Institute for Experimental Orthopaedics
and Dept. of Orthopaedic Surgery,
Saarland University Medical Center,
Saarland University, Homburg, Germany

Bert Mandelbaum
MD
Santa Monica Orthopedic & Sports Medicine Group
Santa Monica, CA, USA

LIST OF CONTRIBUTORS

Fredrik Almqvist
MD, Professor
Orthopaedic Department
Ghent University Hospital
Gent, Belgium

Jason Boyer
MD
Santa Monica Orthopedic & Sports
Medicine Group
Santa Monica, CA, USA

Lorenzo Boldrini
MD
OASI Bioresearch Foundation Gobbi
N.P.O.
Milan, Italy

Mats Brittberg
MD, Professor
Cartilage Research Unit
Orthopaedic Department
Gothenburg University
Kungsbacka, Sweden

Peter U. Brucker
MD
Dept.of Orthopaedic Sports Medicine
Klinikum Rechts der Isar
University of Munich
Munich, Germany

Magali Cucchiarini
PhD, Priv.-Doz.
Institute for Experimental Orthopaedics
Saarland University
Homburg, Germany

Marco Delcogliano
MD
Orthopaedic and Traumatology Dept.
San Carlo di Nancy Hospital
Roma, Italy

Daniela Deponti
PhD
Department of Sport, Nutrition and
Health Sciences
University of Milan, Italy

Aad Dhollander
MD
Orthopaedic Department
Ghent University Hospital
Gent, Belgium

Jaroslaw Deszczynski
MD,PhD
Warsaw Medical University
Warsaw, Poland

Alessandro Di Martino
MD
III Orthopaedic Clinic – Biomechanics
Laboratory
Istituto Ortopedico Rizzoli
Bologna, Italy

Matej Drobnic
MD, PhD, Assistant Professor
Dept. of Orthopaedic Surgery
University Medical Centre Ljubljana
Ljubljana, Slovenia

Milan Držík
PhD
Department of Applied Optics
International Laser Centre
Bratislava, Slovakia

Joao Espregueira-Mendes
MD
Clínica Saude Atlântica Estádio do
Dragão
Porto, Portugal

Giuseppe Filardo
MD
III Orthopaedic Clinic – Biomechanics
Laboratory
Istituto Ortopedico Rizzoli
Bologna, Italy

Pierre-Jean Françin
PhD
UMR-CNRS 7561 Physiopathologie,
Pharmacologie et Ingénierie du
cartilage
Université Henri Poincaré
Nancy, France

Pascale Gegout
PhD
UMR-CNRS 7561 Physiopathologie,
Pharmacologie et Ingénierie du
cartilage
Université Henri Poincaré
Nancy, France

Pierre Gillet
MD, Professor
UMR-CNRS 7561 Physiopathologie,
Pharmacol
ogie et Ingénierie du cartilage
Université Henri Poincaré
Nancy, France

Giovanni Giordano
MD
III Orthopaedic Clinic – Biomechanics
Laboratory
Istituto Ortopedico Rizzoli
Bologna, Italy

Alberto Gobbi
MD
OASI Bioresearch Foundation Gobbi
N.P.O.
Milan, Italy

Milan Handl
MD, PhD, Professor
Orthopaedic Clinic
University Hospital Motol
Prague, Czech Republic

Didier Hannouche
MD, PhD, Professor
Department of Orthopaedic Surgery
Laboratoire de Recherches
Orthopédiques
CNRS, Université Paris 7
Paris, France

Andreas Imhoff
MD, Professor
Dept. of Orthopaedic Sports Medicine
Klinikum Rechts der Isar
University of Munich
Munich, Germany

Gunnar Knutsen
MD, PhD
Head of Orthopaedic department
University Hospital North-Norway
Tromsoe, Norway

Elizaveta Kon
MD
III Orthopaedic Clinic – Biomechanics
Laboratory
Istituto Ortopedico Rizzoli
Bologna, Italy

Delphine Logeart-Avramoglou
PhD
Laboratoire de Recherches
Orthopédiques
CNRS, Université Paris 7
Paris, France

Henning Madry
MD, Professor
Institute for Experimental Orthopaedics
and Dept. of Orthopaedic Surgery,
Saarland University Medical Center,
Saarland University, Homburg, Germany

Didier Mainard
MD, Professor
UMR-CNRS 7561 Physiopathologie,
Pharmacologie et Ingénierie du
cartilage
Université Henri Poincaré
Nancy, France

Bert Mandelbaum
MD
Santa Monica Orthopedic & Sports
Medicine Group
Santa Monica, CA, USA

Laura Mangiavini
MD
Residency Program in Orthopaedics and
Traumatology,
University of Milano-Bicocca
Italy

Maurilio Marcacci
MD, Professor
III Orthopaedic Clinic – Biomechanics
Laboratory
Istituto Ortopedico Rizzoli
Bologna, Italy

Giulio Maria Marcheggiani Muccioli
MD
III Orthopaedic Clinic – Biomechanics
Laboratory
Istituto Ortopedico Rizzoli
Bologna, Italy

Stefan Marlovits
MD, Professor
Dept. of Traumatology
University of Vienna
Vienna, Austria

Giuliana Niceforo
MD
Orthopaedic Department
Catania University
Catania, Italy

Jochen Paul
MD
Dept. of Orthopaedic Sports Medicine
Klinikum Rechts der Isar
University of Munich
Munich, Germany

Giuseppe Peretti
MD
Orthopaedics and Traumatology Dept.
San Raffaele Scientific Institute
Milan, Italy

Hervé Petite
PhD
Laboratoire de Recherches
Orthopédiques
CNRS, Université Paris 7
Paris, France

Nathalie Presle
PhD
UMR-CNRS 7561 Physiopathologie,
Pharmacologie et Ingénierie du
cartilage
Université Henri Poincaré
Nancy, France

Giovanni Ravazzolo
MD
Unit of Radiology and Diagnostic
Imaging
Istituto Ortopedico Rizzoli
Bologna, Italy

James Richardson
MD
Institute of Orthopaedics
Robert Jones & Agnes Hunt
Orthopaedic Hospital
Oswestry, UK

May Arna Risberg
PT, PhD
Professor and chairman
NAR, Norwegian School of Sport
Sciences
Orthopaedic Dept., University Hospital
Oslo, Norway

Ines Sherifi
MD
Laboratoire de Recherches
Orthopédiques
CNRS, Université Paris 7
Paris, France

Konrad Slynarski
MD, PhD
Sports Medicine Center CMS
Warsaw, Poland

Siegfried Trattnig
MD, Professor
Dept. of Radiology
University of Vienna
Vienna, Austria

Dieter Van Assche
PT, PhD
Dept. of Musculoskeletal Sciences
University Hospital Leuven
Leuven, Belgium

Ferdinand Varga
PhD
Department of Biophysics
Charles University, 2nd Faculty of
Medicine
Prague, Czech Republic

Peter Verdonk
MD, PhD
Orthopaedic Department
Ghent University Hospital
Gent, Belgium

René Verdonk
MD, PhD, Prof
Orthopaedic Department
Ghent University Hospital
Gent, Belgium

Stephan Vogt
MD, Associate Professor
Dept. of Orthopaedic Sports Medicine
Klinikum Rechts der Isar
University of Munich
Munich, Germany

Goetz Welsch
MD
Department of Radiology
University of Vienna
Vienna, Austria

Barbara Wondrasch
PT
Vienna Sports Medicine Center
Vienna, Austria

Stefano Zaffagnini
MD
III Orthopaedic Clinic – Biomechanics
Laboratory
Istituto Ortopedico Rizzoli
Bologna, Italy

Viviana Zarbà
MD
Orthopaedic and Traumatology Dept.
Sant'Elia Hospital
Caltanissetta, Italy

CONTENTS

PREFACE

The art of medicine cannot be inherited, nor can it be copied from books....
Paracelsus

It is quite well-known that cartilage when injured is difficult to repair. However, the last 20 years have been stimulating as the era of tissue engineering has opened up a stronger collaboration between basic science and clinical research in order to improve the repair of injured cartilage.
In Porto, 2008, the ESSKA Cartilage Committee presented a symposium on cartilage related problems including both basic and clinical research and clinical problems. Based on those presentations and with help from DJO Publishing we decided to put together the presentations into chapters for a book on current concepts of cartilage repair.

This book is the first in a series on cartilage related matters that hopefully will be useful for surgeons and basic scientists working on treating patients with cartilage injuries. We are very grateful to all authors that have contributed to make this book complete with updates of current concepts. We are also very grateful to DJO for making this publication possible.
One detail has been very obvious; the authors have all been very enthusiastic to take part in writing their chapters which has been stimulating for the editors. We hope that the readers will be stimulated as well to learn more about cartilage for the benefit of our patients.

"Always laugh when you can. It is cheap medicine." - Lord Byron

The Editors

"Formerly, when religion was strong and science weak, men mistook magic for medicine; now, when science is strong and religion weak, men mistake medicine for magic."

(Thomas Szasz; The Second Sin, 1973)

Chapter 1.

Basic Science of Articular Cartilage Repair

Giuseppe M. Peretti, Laura Mangiavini, Daniela Deponti

Take Home Message

- *Articular cartilage is a complex tissue having extraordinary biomechanical properties which are dependent on the particular composition and structure.*
- *Once damaged, the articular cartilage is unable to initiate a spontaneous and efficient regenerative process.*
- *When the lesion reaches the subchondral bone, mesenchymal stem cells together with the blood clot are able to fill the defect and begin to produce some of the macromolecules of the native articular cartilage, such as collagen type II and proteoglycans but also collagen type I. Nevertheless, the reparative cells fail to organize the molecules into a normal layered organized structure. This usually leads to a long-term failure of the reparative tissue.*

Cartilage morphology

Adult articular cartilage is a tissue of mesenchymal origin that covers the articulating surfaces of bones and is capable of maintaining its properties for decades. Articular cartilage has different functions: it spreads the applied load onto the subchondral bone; it provides the articular surfaces with low friction and lubrication; it is also responsible for the mechanism of shock-absorption.

The main component of articular cartilage is water that forms 65 to 80% of the total weight; the dry weight is composed of 45% type II collagen, the 35% is represented by proteoglycans and the remaining part of the dry weight is composed of glycoproteins and cells. In the adult cartilaginous tissue, the cells represent less than 10% of total volume. Cartilage is an avascular, aneural and alymphatic tissue; therefore chondrocytes receive nutrients by diffusion from the synovial tissue.

Morphologically, articular cartilage can be divided into four zones (Fig. 1): the superficial zone which represents the 10-20% of the full thickness, the transitional or middle zone which fills the 40-60% of the tissue, the deep zone which occupies the 30% of the full thickness and the calcified cartilage zone. This is a thin layer of tissue right above the subchondral bone, which, in turn, is composed by the cortical endplate, a thin layer of cortical haversian bone, and by the trabecular spongy bone. At the board between the deep zone and the calcified cartilage, a thin line called tide mark can be identified, considered a crucial structure in the load transfer from the cartilage to the underlying bone[1,3].

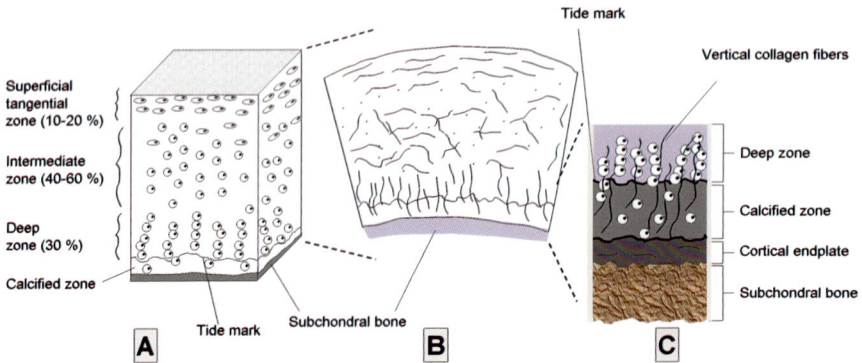

Figure 1: Schematic draw of the different layers of the articular cartilage, showing the distribution of the cells (A), of the collagen fibers (B) and the detail of the osteocartilaginous passage (C).

The distribution and the functions of the extracellular matrix and the chondrocytes are different in these regions: in the superficial area, the collagen fibrils are disposed parallel to the surface, the chondrocytes are elongated and they synthesize high concentration of collagen and low concentration of proteoglycan; additionally, the water content is at the highest level. In the transitional zone, the collagen fibers are randomly disposed and the proteoglycans' concentration is higher. In the deep zone, the water content is at the lowest level, while the proteoglycans are at their highest concentration; moreover, the collagen fibers are arranged perpendicularly to the joint surface and round-shaped chondrocytes form columns having the same direction of the collagen fibers. At this level, thick collagen fibers go across the tide mark, allowing a stable union between the deep layer and the calcified cartilage[13]. In the calcified cartilage zone, the chondrocytes express a hypertrophic phenotype, being embedded in a calcified matrix.

The extracellular matrix composition varies together with its proximity to the chondrocyte. As a matter of fact, the matrix surrounding a single cell, called pericellular matrix, is rich in proteoglycans and type VI collagen; the territorial matrix surrounds the pericellular region of a single chondrocyte and is comprised within a cluster of cells including their pericellular matrix. In the deep zone, it surrounds each single column of cells. This matrix is rich both of proteoglycans and collagen type II fibers. The interterritorial matrix forms most of the volume of all types of matrices, made of proteoglycans and the largest diameter of collagen fibrils[1].

Cartilage components and biomechanics

The biomechanical properties of articular cartilage are supported by the two main components of the extracellular matrix: the proteoglycans and the type II collagen fibers. Both these macromolecules form a complex network which allows for loading of the body weight for many decades.

Type II collagen is typical of the articular cartilage and represents more than 95% of the total weight of collagen in this tissue; other types of collagen present in cartilage are V, VI, IX, X and XI. Collagen fibers in cartilage are thinner than those present in other tissues like bone or tendons. In fact, the mean diameter of a type II collagen varies from a minimum of 10 to a maximum of 100 nanometers. The main characteristic of a collagen fibril is the triple helical structure, where a single molecule is folded with two others. The collagen triple helix is formed by the union of three chains called alpha chains which have a sequence rich in glycine (33%) and proline (25%); the alpha helix is composed by a repetition of a sequence that can be represented as Gly-Xaa-Yaa, where most of the time Xaa is proline and Yaa is frequently occupied by hydroxiproline or hydroxilisine. Thanks to the presence of glycine, the other aminoacids are exposed out of the helix. The proline is responsible of the left-handed spiral shape of the protein complex while hydroxiproline (or hydroxilisine) gives stability to the triple helix. This complex structure gives to type II collagen fibers an incredible resistance to traction forces[5].

The other collagens in the extracellular matrix are thought to give more stability to the type II fibrils, like for example type XI collagen that is not assembled into fibrils but forms covalent cross-links between two or more fibrils of collagen type II.

The main cartilage proteoglycan is the aggrecan, which is formed by a "core" protein bound to others molecules called glycosaminoglycans (GAGs); the most represented GAGs are keratin sulphate and chondroitin sulphate, which consist of long unbranched chains of disaccharide units. The core protein is linked to a molecule of hyaluronic acid by other proteins that form the "linking complex". A single bundle of hyaluronic acid is capable of linking several aggrecan molecules. These macromolecules have repeating carboxyl (COOH) and/or sulphate (SO_4) groups, which, in solution, become ionized (COO^- and SO_3^-). In the physiologic environment, they require positive counterions such as Ca^{2+} and Na^+ to maintain overall electroneutrality. These ions within the interstitial water increase the Donnan osmotic pressure effect, and, ultimately, allow for the attraction of water inside the tissue. Therefore, the tissue considerably increases volume, which is eventually limited by the presence of the collagen fibrils. With aging, the number of GAGs founded in this complex decreases and, therefore, also the number of negative charges diminishes[10].

The biomechanical properties of articular cartilage have been studied with different models. The most suitable for the cartilaginous matrix seems to be the biphasic model proposed by Mow twenty years ago[7]. In his model the response to various stresses is determined by an interaction between a solid phase, represented by the matrix and a liquid phase, represented by water.

The complex network, formed by proteoglycans and type II collagen, provides the articular cartilage with two characteristics: the resistance to a compressive stress and the high elasticity. The network confers to the matrix a porosity of 60 Amstrongs in normal conditions, which could be reduced up to 20 Amstrongs when cartilage is compressed. When a load is applied, the water flows very slowly out of the tissue. This slow flow is due both to the low porosity and to the presence of the negative charges contained in the GAGs molecules, which exert a strong resistance to a volume reduction. In these conditions, the main responsible for the load bearing is represented by the liquid: the uncompressible water sustains the compressive stresses, ultimately protecting the solid components of the cartilage matrix, which appears only partially involved in the biomechanical response. This is the so called flow-dependent resistance to a compressive stress. However, if cartilage is damaged, such as in osteoarthritis, the water flows out rapidly from the extracellular matrix involving significantly the solid component of the tissue in the biomechanical response. This may lead to a rapid deterioration of the whole cartilaginous tissue[11].

On the other hand, when a shear force is applied, no interstitial fluid flow occurs and the tissue generally deforms thanks to the randomly organized collagen fibers of the transitional zone. In these conditions, the solid matrix is directly involved in the biomechanical response and, therefore, is exposed to deterioration. In order to reduce the shear forces, the cartilage tissue optimizes the superficial lubrication by a morphologically and biochemically perfectly organized structure and by the presence of the synovial fluid inside the joint. Again, any type of damage, which causes an increase of the shear forces, like the superficial fibrillation, may lead to an increase of the involvement of the solid matrix in the biomechanical response and, therefore, to a tissue deterioration.

Articular cartilage does not regenerate

Articular cartilage is a metabolically active tissue, but it has a poor intrinsic healing potential when damaged. As a matter of fact, traumatic lesions and degenerative diseases strongly affect joint function, as the reparative process of articular cartilage frequently results in fibrous tissue. This reparative tissue has different biochemical composition and inferior biomechanical properties compared to those of hyaline cartilage. Besides, articular cartilage is able to repair but not to regenerate itself. In fact, a reparative process may replace the damaged cartilage by a tissue that fails in the restoring of the original properties of the native matrix[4]. The cartilage response to traumas is limited for two main reasons: first, cartilage is an avascularized tissue and, therefore, when a cartilaginous lesion occurs, the blood clot formation can not take place and the inflammation response, often accompanied by the migration of the undifferentiated cells to the lesion site, is absent. Second, it lacks of undifferentiated cells. In fact, the highly differentiated chondrocyte is the only cellular type present in cartilage, having limited synthetic and mitotic potential[15]. Additionally, the number of the chondrocytes and their synthetic properties further decline with age, making the repair process further difficult in adult and old patients.

Different lesions lead to different responses

Hyaline cartilage could be subjected to different types of lesions, which may lead to different repair responses. Generally, cartilage lesion can be divided into superficial lesions, blunt traumas and subchondral bone injuries.
Superficial lesions (partial thickness defects). The superficial zone of hyaline cartilage consists of flattened chondrocytes and tightly packed type II collagen fibers oriented parallel to the articular surface. This layer is believed to provide resistance to shear forces and protect the deeper layers. The damage starts with collagen fibrillation at the top of the articular surface. In this stage, the histological proteoglycan specific stain (safranin-o) diminishes as a result of the lack of proteoglycans. Chondrocytes proliferate in clusters and start to produce a large amount of proteoglycans, but they don't migrate nor fill the defect; the newly synthesized proteoglycans remain at the neighborhood of the chondrocytes clusters. Moreover, a superficial lesion increases the permeability of the tissue and increases the direct biomechanical response of the macromolecular framework during compression.
The superficial layer acts also as a barrier between the synovial fluid and the cartilage isolating the chondrocytes from the immune system[14]. Moreover, as cartilage is an avascular tissue, the damaged site could not be reached by neither inflammatory nor undifferentiated cells from the bone marrow. Mesenchymal stem cells from the synovial membrane, however, could migrate across the articular surface into the lesion, but cartilage contains proteoglycans which confer antiadhesive properties to the tissue, thereby inhibiting the attachment of the cells to the extracellular matrix[2]. In fact, these migrated cells could be experimentally entrapped in the reparative site by the enzymatic neutralization of the proteoglycan (Fig.2)

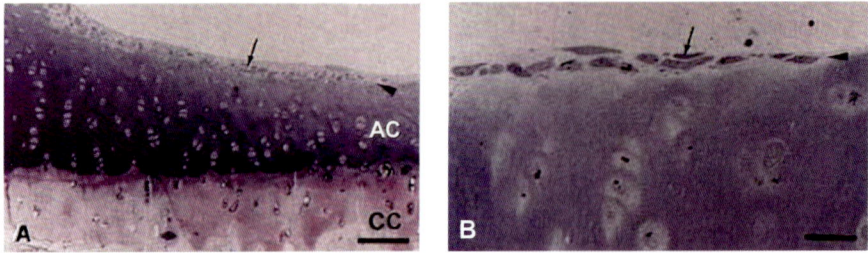

Figure 2: Photomicrograph of semithin sections (stained with toluidine blue) from a partial-thickness defect treated with chondroitinase ABC. After four weeks, a continuous mantle of mesenchymal cells (arrow, A) is visible, consisting of one to several layers (arrow, B), along the surface of the defect. AC = articular cartilage and CC = calcified cartilage. The arrowheads denote the interface between host and repair tissue (A: x 120, bar = 80 micrometers; B: x 475, bar = 20 micrometers). Published with permission by J Bone Joint Surg Am (reference # 2).

If the damage progresses, fragments of articular cartilage may be released into the joint and the subchondral bone may be exposed. As a result, the load is directly transmitted to the underlying subchondral bone, which responses by increasing its density and thickness.

Blunt trauma. A single or multiple high load shocks or repetitive lower load traumas could cause a chondral lesion without the visible alteration of the superficial area. In particular, in a blunt trauma, the load is transmitted throughout the whole thickness of the tissue up to the deepest layers; the osteochondral bone reacts and becomes progressively thicker. This could cause a reduction of the shock absorber effect at this level, eventually leading to the deterioration of the above cartilage layers[9]. To this end, studies in animal models on the etiopathogenesis of the arthrosis have demonstrated that the alteration of the subchondral bone may precede those of the superficial layers[8]. Moreover, great impact stresses may cause the rupture of the thick collagen fibers which go across the tide mark. This event severely interferes with the load transmission at this level and may lead to a progressive degeneration of the whole cartilage. Furthermore, in vitro and in vivo studies have demonstrated that blunt traumas result also in injury to chondrocytes[6] (Fig. 3).

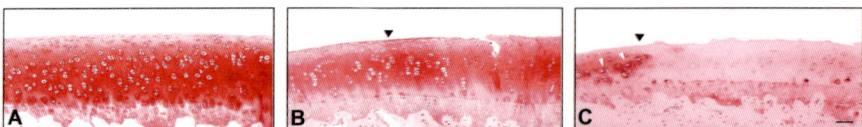

Figure 3: Histological sections (stained with safranin 0) of femoral condyles from the in vivo impaction study. Solid black arrows indicate border between the impacted region on the right side and adjacent nonimpacted region on the left side. A, contralateral control condyle. B, impacted condyles showing superficial roughening and cracks up to 20% of the thickness at the time of the trauma. C, condyles at 3 weeks after impaction have significant proteoglycan and chondrocyte loss through

out the entire depth in the impacted region. Chondrocytes adjacent to the impacted site appear to be synthesizing PG as indicated by the intense red staining around the cells (white arrow). Scale bar is 50 micrometers. Published with permission by J Orthop Trauma (reference # 6).

The apoptosis of the chondrocytes and thereby the disturbance of cartilage matrix turnover may ultimately result in long-term disruption of the cartilage structure and interference with the biomechanical function.

Osteochondral lesions. This type of damage consists in a full thickness cartilage defect extending into the underlying subchondral bone. These lesions are therefore accessible to bone marrow cells, such as blood cells, macrophages and mesenchymal stem cells. Following damage, a fibrin clot is rapidly formed in the defect and in the bony part of the lesion; then, after few days, mesenchymal stem cells migrate from the bone marrow to the periphery of the blood clot and start to differentiate into chondrocytes and osteoblasts in the bony part and, in few weeks, they fill the defect. Under the stimulation of local growth factors, these cells start to produce collagen type II but also collagen type I, and the macromolecules of the native articular cartilage. However, these are less than those of the normal cartilage and the reparative cells fail to organize the molecules into a normally organized layered structure. Moreover, in this reparative process, the superficial zone is often only partially restored. The reparative tissue, therefore, possesses properties that are intermediate between the cartilaginous and the fibrous tissue and does not restore the normal structure, composition, and mechanical properties of the hyaline cartilage[1]. As a consequence, in the long term, a process of degeneration starts and leads to failure of the reparative tissue. In fact, while the bony integration is efficient, histological aspect of the area between the reparative cartilage and the native tissue often shows discontinuity between the two regions: articular cartilage is rich of proteoglycans, which have antiadhesive properties impeding the appropriate bonding of the two components. Furthermore, the native cartilage around the damaged area is often necrotic and remains inert without remodeling phenomena[12] (Fig. 4).

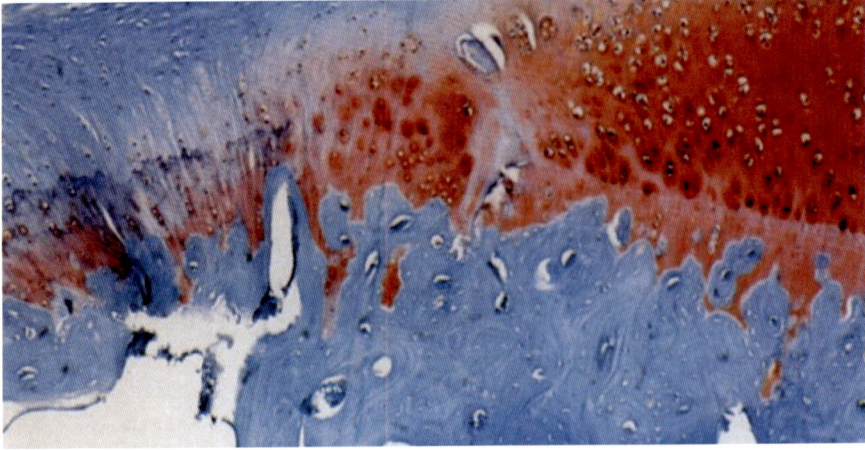

Figure 4: Photomicrograph (stained with safranin 0), made forty-eight weeks after creation of a defect in a rabbit repair model, showing repair tissue at the left and residual articular cartilage at the right. Considerable degeneration of the repair tissue is visible, consisting in almost exclusively fibrous nature. This region is also hypocellular. Fissures, which indicate of a poor mechanical stability, are present at the upper left. Published with permission by J Orthop Trauma (reference # 12).

The healing process of the osteochondral lesions is influenced by different factors: the size and the location of the damaged area and the age of the patient. In fact, extensive defects or lesions in the weight-bearing areas have minor chances for successful healing. On the other hand, young patients have a better response to osteochondral lesions having a more effective synthesis of macromolecules; moreover, young articular cartilage still presents some vascularization, thereby allowing for a better cellular response to the injury.

Conclusions

The biochemical composition and the morphological organization of the articular cartilage are fundamental for the correct biomechanical function of this tissue. In physiological conditions, the extracellular matrix and the joint environment allow the cartilage tissue for a biomechanical response with practically no tissue consumption and degradation. However, when a lesion occurs, the remaining cells are not able to organize an adequate regenerative response or, in case of an osteochondral lesion, the infiltrating cells fail in the attempt of organizing the newly formed tissue into a biomechanically functional matrix. Therefore, especially in large lesion involving weight-bearing areas in adult patients, this leads to a long-term failure of the reparative tissue, making the defect of the articular cartilage one of the most problematic and challenging issue for the orthopaedic surgeon.

References

1. Bhosale AM; Richardson JB, Articular cartilage: structure, injuries and review of management, Br Med Bul, 2008, 87:77-95

2. Hunziker EB; Rosenberg LC, Repair of partial-thickness defects in articular cartilage: cell recruitment from the synovial membrane, J Bone Joint Surg Am, 1996, 78:721-33

3. Imhof H; Sulzbacher I; Grampp S; Czerny C; Youssefzadeh S; Kainberger F, Subchondral bone and cartilage disease: a rediscovered functional unit, Invest Radiol, 2000, 35:581-588

4. Khan IM; Gilbert SJ; Singhrao SK; Duance VC; Archer CW, Cartilage integration: evaluation of the reasons for failure of integration during cartilage repair. A review, Eur Cell Mater, 2008, 16:26-39

5. Kolàcnà L; Bakesovà J; Varga F; Kostàkovà E; Plankà L; Necas A; Lukàs D; Amler E; Pelouch V, Biochemical and biophysical aspects of collagen nanostructure in the extreacellular matrix, Physiol Res ,2007, 56 Suppl 1:S51-60

6. Milentijevic D; Rubel IF; Liew AS; Helfet DL; Torzilli PA, An in vivo rabbit model for cartilage trauma: a preliminary study of the influence of impact stress magnitude on chondrocyte death and matrix damage, J Orthop Trauma, 2005, 19:466-73

7. Mow VC; Kuei SC; Lai WM; Armstrong CG, Bifasic creep and stress relaxation of articular cartilagein compression: theory and experiments, J Biomech Eng, 1980, 102:73-84

8. Muraoka T; Hagino H; Okano T; Enokida M; Teshima R, Role of subchondral bone in osteoarthritis development: a comparative study of two strains of guinea pigs with and without spontaneously occurring osteoarthritis, Arthritis Rheum, 2007, 56:3366-3374

9. Pugh JW; Rose RM; Radin EL, A structural model for the mechanical behavior of trabecular bone, J Biomech, 1973, 6:657-770

10. Roughley PJ, The structure and functions of cartilage proteoglycans, Europ Cells Mat, 2006, 12:92-101

11. Samuels J; Krasnokutsky S; Abramson SB, Osteoarthritis: a tale of three tissues, Bull NYU Hosp Jt Dis, 2008, 66:244-250

12. Shapiro F; Koide S; Glimcher MJ, Cell origin and differentiation in the repair of full-thickness defects of articular cartilage, J Bone Joint Surg Am, 1993, 75:532-553

13. Shirazi R; Shirazi-Adl A; Hurtig M, Role of cartilage collagen fibrils networks in knee joint biomechanics under compression, J Biomech, 2008, 41:3340-3348

14. Simon TM; Jackson DW, Articular cartilage: injury pathways and treatment options, Sports Med Arthrosc, 2006, 14:146-154

15. Stubbs AJ; Potter HG, Section VII: Chondral lesions, J Bone Joint Surg Am, 2009, 91 Suppl 1:119

16. Walker JM, Pathomechanics and classification of cartilage lesions, facilitation of repair, J Orthop Sports Phys Ther, 1998, 28:216-231

"The art of medicine cannot be inherited, nor can it be copied from books..."

(Paracelsus)

CHAPTER 2.

CELL REQUIREMENTS AND CULTURE CONDITIONS FOR CARTILAGE REPAIR

Didier Hannouche, Ines Sherifi,
Delphine Logeart-Avramoglou, Hervé Petite

Take Home Message

Three factors play a crucial role in the chondrocytic differentiation process:
1. The growth factors
2. Oxygen conditions during the culture process
3. The nature and the size of mechanical loads applied during culture
These factors must be optimised before considering a possible clinical application.

Introduction

Three major strategies are currently being studied to repair cartlage defects with competent cells: (i) the implantaton of culture expanded cells seeded onto bio-degradable scaffolds; (ii) the implantion of a more or less pre-shaped and struc-tured tissue, obtained in vitro by the assembly and three-dimensional culture of cells and a resorbable matrix; (iii) the stimulation of in situ tissue repair by differ-ent means, including growth factors or genetically modified cells.

Several cell sources are available to manufacture cartilage structures with a biochemical composition and mechanical properties that are close to that of native cartilage. Historically, chondrocytes were first proposed to repair cartilage defects for their natural capacity to produce a hyaline cartilage matrix rich in glycosaminoglycans and type II collagen. Another important source of chondrogenic cells is the bone marrow, a natural reservoir of multipotent cells, referred to as mesenchymal stem cells (MSC), that have the potential to differentiate in vitro into chondrocytes under specific culture conditions. A number of parameters may determine the chondrogenic differentiation process of MSC and will be discussed in this chapter: the nature of the three-dimensional matrix, the need for a bioreactor culture system, and the choice and sequence of growth factors administration.

1 - Obtaining the right scaffold

1.1- Material specifications
A number of materials have been suggested to induce chondrogenesis (synthetic polymers, collagen, hyaluronic acid, fibrin, gelatin, alginate...). These are three-dimensional matrices that provide a permissive environment, allow cell-to-cell contact, inhibit cell dedifferentiation, and stimulate the redifferentiation of chondrocytes[33]. Combined with stem cells, they enhance the initial condensation phase, cell proliferation and their differentiation into chondrocytes. Such substratum should have specific biochemical (i.e., molecules of the extracellular matrix), physicochemical (such as surface free energy, charge, hydrophobicity) as well as geometric aspects (for example, three dimensional (3D), interconnected porosity)[34].
Scaffolds for cartilage engineering should satisfy a number of criteria. Such matrices should be: (i) biocompatible, i.e., non-immunogenic and non-toxic; (ii) absorbable (with rates of resorption commensurate to those of cartilage formation); (iii) easy to manufacture and sterilize; and (vi) easy to handle in the surgery room, preferably without preparatory procedures (in order to limit the risk of infection). The following macro- and micro-structural properties of biomaterial scaffolds are critical for optimal cell ingrowth:

- Porosity
Three-dimensional scaffolds for cartilage tissue regeneration require internal microarchitecture, specifically highly porous interconnected structures and a large surface-to-volume ratios, to promote cell in-growth and cell distribution throughout the matrix. Pore sizes in the range of 200-900 µm have performed most satisfactorily in these applications.

- Topography and surface chemistry
Particle size, shape, and surface roughness affect cellular adhesion, proliferation, and phenotype. Specifically, cells are sensitive and responsive to the chemistry, topography and surface energy of the material substrates with which they interact. In this respect, the type, amount and conformation of specific proteins which adsorb onto materials surfaces, subsequently modulate cell functions. With re-

gards to cartigae formation, the presence of negative electrostatic charges at a density of 2-10/ nm^2 would be beneficial for cell adhesion and proliferation[34].

1.2- Scaffolds for cartilage engineering

Polymers (either naturally-derived or synthetic ones) are an important category of materials for cartilage tissue engineering applications.

Natural polymers are extracted from animal and vegetable sources. These compounds are of major interest in tissue engineering since they are biocompatible, biodegradable and natural substrates onto which cells can adhere, proliferate, and function. Additionally, such material substrates can be prepared in various forms including strips, sheets, sponges and beads.

Synthetic polymeric materials, free of potential contamination, have proven useful and are used to develop biocompatible substrates tailored for specific medical applications. One of the polymers that has been considered for potential use in cartilage repair is the polyglycolic acid (PGA) polymer and its homopolymer derivatives. Various chemical techniques were investigated and were successful in developing three-dimensional porous structures that can be custom-designed to the size and shape of the patient's defect. The most widely used processing method for polymeric scaffolds involves solution-cast/particulate-leaching to tailor three-dimensional porous structures. Recent advances in computer technology enabled development of new fabrication, such as rapid prototyping (RP) techniques, for use in the tissue-engineering field. RP techniques utilize layered manufacturing approaches, whereby 3D objects are fabricated layer by layer via processing of solid sheet, liquid or powder material stocks.

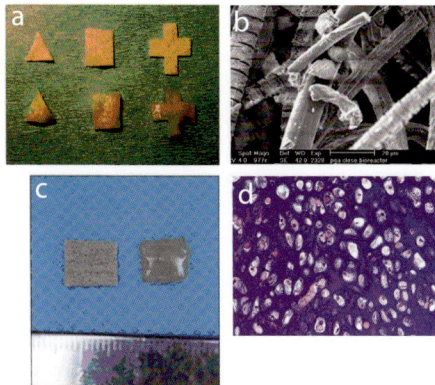

Figure 1: Chondrocytes were seeded onto PGA scaffolds (Fig 1a) and cultured in the bioreactor for 6 weeks. Scanning electron microscopy showed homogeneous distribution and adhesion of cells on the scaffold (Fig 1b). Fig 1c shows a PGA/chondrocytes construct at 6 weeks, and Fig 1d shows the presence of a cartilaginous extracellular matrix throughout the section (toluidine blue staining).

2- Cell source

2.1- Chondrocytes

The repair of tissue loss by the differentiated cells in the articular cartilage is an attractive solution at first sight and was suggested by several authors with different biomaterials:

- These may include collagen sponges in the Novocart® (TETEC, Reutlingen, Germany) and Chondrokin® (Orthogen, Düsseldorf, Germany) products, or collagen gel in the CaReS® (Fraunhofer Institute for Interfacial Engineering and Biotechnology, Stuttgart) and Atelocollagen® (Koken, Japan) products.

- In the Cartipatch® process, the chondrocytes are seeded in alginate supplemented with agarose (Cartipatch®, TBF, France). Recently, a phase II multicentre clinical study was conducted on 17 patients presenting with traumatic lesions or osteochondritis of the knee[43]. The IKDC score was significantly improved, while the histology analysis performed in 13 cases revealed an essentially hyaline-like cartilage in 8 cases. MRI performed at 2 years showed a signal that was identical to the normal cartilage in 10 out of 15 cases. A comparative study versus mosaicplasty is ongoing.

- Finally, chondrocytes may be supplemented with hyaluronic acid. Nehrer[38] recently reported the results of 36 symptomatic patients treated with Hyalograft C® (Fidia, Italy). The best results were obtained in patients under 30 years with a single condyle lesion. The results seemed to be maintained at 3-years follow-up. Despite these encouraging results, the use of chondrocytes as a cell source for cartilage engineering raises a number of issues. The amount of chondrocytes in the articular cartilage is relatively low, their proliferation potential is limited and the harvest itself requires an additional surgical procedure with its potential complications. In addition, expansion of chondrocytes on a plastic monolayer cell culture leads to chondrocyte dedifferentiation with a reduction in the expression of phenotypic markers, such as type II, IX, XI collagen and aggrecan. Cells cultured in such conditions adopt a fibroblastic shape and secrete type I and III collagen[4, 20]. Finally, the proliferation potential of chondrocytes is variable depending on the donor age and site, which limits the relevance of this procedure for cartilage repair in adults[12].

2.2- Mesenchymal stem cells

Bone marrow, a natural repository of skeletal stem cells, has been used as the source of cartilage progenitor cells. When plated at low cell densities, the cells form pluripotent fibroblastic colonies clonal in origin which were initially referred to as "colony-forming units-fibroblasts" (CFU-F). They represent a small (0.001-0.01%) fraction of the total population of the nucleated cells present in marrow and are now known as "mesenchymal stem cells" (MSCs)[5-7, 24, 41]. The progeny of MSCs are "bone marrow stromal fibroblasts" (BMSFs). Under appropriate experimental in vitro conditions, MSCs can differentiate into bone, cartilage, adipose tissue and hematopoietic-supportive stroma cells[50]. The chondrogenic differentiation of MSC is dependent on a strong transcription factor (Sox 9)[10], and requires specific culture conditions. It is encouraged by three-dimensional culture systems, and the addition of Dexamethasone, ascorbic acid and Transforming Growth Factor β (TGFβ)[23] in a culture medium devoid of fetal bovine serum (FBS)[28].

From the cartilage tissue engineering perspective, MSCs have a number of advantages: (i) their isolation is easy as it relies primarily on the ability of these cells to adhere to tissue-culture plastic; (ii) they have a high proliferative potential which can be maintained up to 26 culture passages. In fact, it has been determined that almost half a billion cells could be obtained at passage 6 even when starting with 100-500 adherent MSCs[17]; (iii) cartilage formation is not correlated to the number of cell passages as long as the human stem cells retain their proliferative potential; and (v) freezing conditions do not affect the potential of MSCs, a condition that greatly facilitates their storage.

Cell sources other than bone marrow have been suggested for the harvest of adult stem cells, in particular fat tissue (subcutaneous fat, and the retropatellar fat pad)[2,18], the synovial membrane[44], peripheral blood[25,26], umbilical cord blood[29], vessels[9,11], and the teeth[37]. Aspiration of peripheral blood appears to be an attractive MSC source, but not all authors have been able to reproduce it[27]. However, before these new sources could be considered as viable alternatives to bone-marrow-derived MSCs, further studies in clinically relevant animal models are needed to better characterize the relative (compared to bone marrow) chondrogenic potential of stem cells isolated from these alternative sources.

To date, use of stem cells in the clinical setting has not been possible in cartilage repair procedures because of pertinent logistics, specifically limitations associated with harvesting bone marrow from the patient and with expanding and differentiating such cells in vitro in short period of time. Additional major hurdles associated with the use of autologous stem cells are: (i) decreased numbers with age; and (ii) variability of the amount and quality of bone marrow aspirations (the source of autologous cells) from patient to patient.

3- Optimal culture conditions for chondrogenic differentiation of MSCs

3.1- Chondrogenic potential of MSC

The possibility of chondrocytic differentiation of MSC was first described on cell pellets[23], and more recently on small-sized supports (<3mm) in gelatin[42], alginate[8], fibrin[40], hyaluronic acid[1], or on nanosupport surfaces[30]. However, the manufacture of small-sized structures that would have enough mechanical properties for clinical applications has until now yielded variable results[19]. Several factors may explain the sometimes contradictory results published in the litterature[35,36]: the species chosen, the initial cell density, the inoculation and culture conditions, and the growth factors used.

3.2- Conditions for the culture of MSC in a bioreactor

Chondrogenic differentiation of MSCs is most often achieved in dynamic three-dimensional culture systems that were developed to preserve the chondrocytic phenotype and avoid the chondrocytic dedifferentiation observed in monolayer cell cultures. Advantages of these 3D culture systems, often referred to as bioreactors, include: (i) a permanent renewal of the culture medium (nutritional requirement and elimination of waste); (ii) a strict control of temperature, pO2 and pH wihin the medium; (iii) the possibility of applying mechanical loading on the constructs during the culture phase; (iv) the establishment of reproducible culture conditions for future clinical applications[48].

The cell seeding step on three-dimensional matrices is a key factor in the manufacture of cartilage structures in vitro. Two parameters significantly influence the quality of the neoformed tissue: the initial cell density, which must be high (>20x106 cells/ml) as it correlates with the production of GAGs and type II collagen[49]; and the uniformity of cell distribution, which determines the final tissue homogeneity[13]. Cell seeding requirements might be achived through bioreactor designs that allow efficient, fast and spatially uniform cell seeding. Medium renewal promotes cell proliferation and enhances the kinetics of cell attachment and differenciation[51]. We recently obtained cartilage tissue from bone marrow derived MSC cultured on PGA scaffolds alone, or supplemented with a type I collagen or alginate gel[16]. Three to six weeks in a bioreactor were necessary to observe the formation of a white, pearly, smooth cartilaginous tissue comparable to that of hyaline cartilage. Histological and immunohistochemical analyses confirmed the presence of a cartilaginous extra-cellular matrix across the entire thickness of the sections. Similar results were also observed with the culture of sheep umbilical cord blood cells seeded on PGA sponges[14]. However, a 12 weeks culture was required to observe a chondrocytic differentiation, and the apposition of a cartilage matrix.

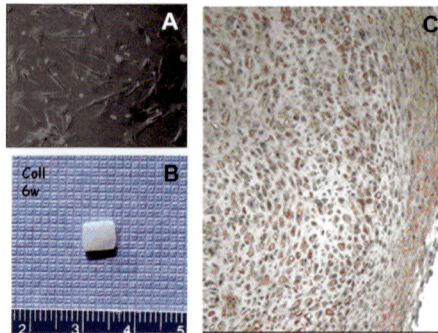

Figure 2: MSCs morphology at day 1 under microscopy (Fig 2a). The thickness of the MSCs seeded constructs increased substantially during time. At 6 weeks, they had a white pearly aspect (Fig 2b). Immunostaining of a 6 weeks PGA-type I collagen/ MSCs construct detected the presence of type II collagen around and within the cells (colorimetrical detection with a labelled streptavidin biotin (LSAB kit).

3.3- Growth factors

Growth factors play an important role in the chondrocytic differentiation of MSC and maintenance of the chondrocytic phenotype. A very large number of factors were studied, specifically the TGFβ, the Insulin-like Growth Factor (IGF), the Fibroblast Growth Factor (FGF), the Platelet-Derived Growth Factor (PDGF), and the Epidermal Growth Factor (EGF). Several studies[15,23,32,39] have focused on the crucial role of TGFβ, FGF 18, and (Bone Morphogenetic Protein 2 (BMP 2), while the IGF, PDGF, and the other FGFs might be efficient only if combined to TGFβ[45]. In vitro, the TGFβ1 and the BMP2 induced an increase in the production of type II collagen and proteoglycans, and a decrease in the production of proteolytic enzymes[21,46]. Nevertheless, it should be highlighted that all these growth factors have a pleiotropic effect and are involved in osteoblast differentiation. Also, contradictory effects of the different growth factors have been described and might be explained by the concentration used, the maturation status of chondrocytes, the species considered, the number of receptors on the cell surface, and the combination or not with another growth factor. For instance, FGF2 is a mitotic factor that stimulates the proliferation of MSC in vitro, while maintaining their chondrocytic differentiation potential[47]. Combined with TGFβ1, it potentiates the effect of TGFβ1 on the differentiation of periosteum cells cultured in alginate cell. The opposite effect is observed when it is combined with TGFβ3[3].

Conclusions

The possibility of repairing osteochondral substance loss with MSC opens up treatment prospects for a large number of patients. The repair of clinically relevant defects will require a very large number of MSC, which in vivo chondrocytic differentiation will probably be incomplete. The in vitro pre-differentiation of MSC into chondrocytes has the advantage of reducing the differentiation of MSC in other phenotypes after implantation, as observed with embryonic stem cells[31]. Finally, due to their relative simplicity, the tissue culture systems that have been developed provide precious information on the chondrocytic differentiation process at a cellular and molecular scale, and help to optimise the in vitro differentiation protocols and the cartilage structure production.

Despite the macroscopic appearance of cartilage fragments obtained in vitro with chondrocytes or MSC, and the presence of a comparable amount of GAGs in the native cartilage, these structures contain a notable amount of type I collagen, and a significantly lower amount of type II collagen than in the native cartilage. Three factors play a crucial role in the chondrocytic differentiation process, and may act independently on the production of GAGs and/or type II collagen[22]: the growth factors, oxygen conditions during the culture process, and the nature and the size of mechanical loads applied during culture. These factors must be optimised before considering a possible clinical application.

Acknowledgement

Part of the work presented in this chapter has been performed in the Laboratory for Tissue Engineering and Organ Fabrication, at Harvard Medical School, Boston, USA (Professor Joseph Vacanti). We are very grateful to Hidetomi Terai, MD, PhD, and Julie Fuchs, MD for their collaboration to this work.

References

1. Angele P, Kujat R, Nerlich M, Yoo J, Goldberg V, Johnstone B. Engineering of osteochondral tissue with bone marrow mesenchymal progenitor cells in a derivatized hyaluronan-gelatin composite sponge. Tissue Eng 1999;5(6):545-54.
2. Awad HA, Wickham MQ, Leddy HA, Gimble JM, Guilak F. Chondrogenic differentiation of adipose-derived adult stem cells in agarose, alginate, and gelatin scaffolds. Biomaterials 2004;25(16):3211-22.
3. Baddoo M, Hill K, Wilkinson R, Gaupp D, Hughes C, Kopen GC, et al. Characterization of mesenchymal stem cells isolated from murine bone marrow by negative selection. J Cell Biochem 2003;89(6):1235-49.
4. Benya PD, Padilla SR. Modulation of the rabbit chondrocyte phenotype by retinoic acid terminates type II collagen synthesis without inducing type I collagen: the modulated phenotype differs from that produced by subculture. Dev Biol 1986;118(1):296-305.
5. Bruder SP, Jaiswal N, Haynesworth SE. Growth kinetics, self-renewal, and the osteogenic potential of purified human mesenchymal stem cells during extensive subcultivation and following cryopreservation. J Cell Biochem 1997;64(2):278-94.
6. Bruder SP, Jaiswal N, Ricalton NS, Mosca JD, Kraus KH, Kadiyala S. Mesenchymal stem cells in osteobiology and applied bone regeneration. Clin Orthop Relat Res 1998(355 Suppl):S247-56.
7. Caplan AI. Review: mesenchymal stem cells: cell-based reconstructive therapy in orthopedics. Tissue Eng 2005;11(7-8):1198-211.
8. Caterson EJ, Nesti LJ, Li WJ, Danielson KG, Albert TJ, Vaccaro AR, et al. Three-dimensional cartilage formation by bone marrow-derived cells seeded in polylactide/alginate amalgam. J Biomed Mater Res 2001;57(3):394-403.
9. De Angelis L, Berghella L, Coletta M, Lattanzi L, Zanchi M, Cusella-De Angelis MG, et al. Skeletal myogenic progenitors originating from embryonic dorsal aorta coexpress endothelial and myogenic markers and contribute to postnatal muscle growth and regeneration. J Cell Biol 1999;147(4):869-78.
10. de Crombrugghe B, Lefebvre V, Behringer RR, Bi W, Murakami S, Huang W. Transcriptional mechanisms of chondrocyte differentiation. Matrix Biol 2000;19(5):389-94.
11. Doherty MJ, Ashton BA, Walsh S, Beresford JN, Grant ME, Canfield AE. Vascular pericytes express osteogenic potential in vitro and in vivo. J Bone Miner Res 1998;13(5):828-38.
12. Dozin B, Malpeli M, Camardella L, Cancedda R, Pietrangelo A. Response of young, aged and osteoarthritic human articular chondrocytes to inflammatory cytokines: molecular and cellular aspects. Matrix Biol 2002;21(5):449-59.
13. Freed LE, Marquis JC, Nohria A, Emmanual J, Mikos AG, Langer R. Neocartilage formation in vitro and in vivo using cells cultured on synthetic biodegradable polymers. J Biomed Mater Res 1993;27(1):11-23.
14. Fuchs JR, Hannouche D, Terada S, Zand S, Vacanti JP, Fauza DO. Cartilage engineering from ovine ombilical cord blood mesenchymal progenitor cells. Stem Cells 2005;23:958-64.
15. Glowacki J, Yates KE, Maclean R, Mizuno S. In vitro engineering of cartilage: effects of serum substitutes, TGF-beta, and IL-1alpha. Orthod Craniofac Res 2005;8(3):200-8.
16. Hannouche D, Terai H, Fuchs JR, Terada S, Zand S, Nasseri BA, et al. Engineering of implantable cartilaginous structures from bone marrow derived mesenchymal stem cells. Tissue Eng 2007 Jan;13(1):87-99.
17. Haynesworth SE, Goshima J, Goldberg VM, Caplan AI. Characterization of cells with osteogenic potential from human marrow. Bone 1992;13(1):81-8.
18. Huang JI, Kazmi N, Durbhakula MM, Hering TM, Yoo JU, Johnstone B. Chondrogenic potential of progenitor cells derived from human bone marrow and adipose tissue: a patient-matched comparison. J Orthop Res 2005;23(6):1383-9.

19. Hunziker EB. Articular cartilage repair: are the intrinsic biological constraints undermining this process insuperable? Osteoarthritis Cartilage 1999;7(1):15-28.

20. Hunziker EB. Articular cartilage repair: basic science and clinical progress. A review of the current status and prospects. Osteoarthritis Cartilage 2002;10(6):432-63.

21. Hunziker EB, Driesang IM, Morris EA. Chondrogenesis in cartilage repair is induced by members of the transforming growth factor-beta superfamily. Clin Orthop Relat Res 2001(391 Suppl):S171-81.

22. Ikenoue T, Trindade MC, Lee MS, Lin EY, Schurman DJ, Goodman SB, et al. Mechanoregulation of human articular chondrocyte aggrecan and type II collagen expression by intermittent hydrostatic pressure in vitro. J Orthop Res 2003;21(1):110-6.

23. Johnstone B, Hering TM, Caplan AI, Goldberg VM, Yoo JU. In vitro chondrogenesis of bone marrow-derived mesenchymal progenitor cells. Exp Cell Res 1998;238(1):265-72.

24. Kadiyala S, Young RG, Thiede MA, Bruder SP. Culture expanded canine mesenchymal stem cells possess osteochondrogenic potential in vivo and in vitro. Cell Transplant 1997;6(2):125-34.

25. Kuwana M, Okazaki Y, Kodama H, Izumi K, Yasuoka H, Ogawa Y, et al. Human circulating CD14+ monocytes as a source of progenitors that exhibit mesenchymal cell differentiation. J Leukoc Biol 2003;74(5):833-45.

26. Kuznetsov SA, Mankani MH, Gronthos S, Satomura K, Bianco P, Robey PG. Circulating skeletal stem cells. J Cell Biol 2001;153(5):1133-40.

27. Lazarus HM, Haynesworth SE, Gerson SL, Caplan AI. Human bone marrow-derived mesenchymal (stromal) progenitor cells (MPCs) cannot be recovered from peripheral blood progenitor cell collections. J Hematother 1997;6(5):447-55.

28. Lee JW, Kim YH, Kim SH, Han SH, Hahn SB. Chondrogenic differentiation of mesenchymal stem cells and its clinical applications. Yonsei Med J 2004;45 Suppl:41-7.

29. Lee OK, Kuo TK, Chen WM, Lee KD, Hsieh SL, Chen TH. Isolation of multipotent mesenchymal stem cells from umbilical cord blood. Blood 2004;103(5):1669-75.

30. Li WJ, Tuli R, Okafor C, Derfoul A, Danielson KG, Hall DJ, et al. A three-dimensional nanofibrous scaffold for cartilage tissue engineering using human mesenchymal stem cells. Biomaterials 2005;26(6):599-609.

31. Mackenzie TC, Flake AW. Multilineage differentiation of human MSC after in utero transplantation. Cytotherapy 2001;3(5):403-5.

32. Majumdar MK, Wang E, Morris EA. BMP-2 and BMP-9 promotes chondrogenic differentiation of human multipotential mesenchymal cells and overcomes the inhibitory effect of IL-1. J Cell Physiol 2001;189(3):275-84.

33. Malda J, van Blitterswijk CA, Grojec M, Martens DE, Tramper J, Riesle J. Expansion of bovine chondrocytes on microcarriers enhances redifferentiation. Tissue Eng 2003;9(5):939-48.

34. Maroudas NG. Sulphonated polystyrene as an optimal substratum for the adhesion and spreading of mesenchymal cells in monovalent and divalent saline solutions. J Cell Physiol 1977;90(3):511-9.

35. Martin I, Padera RF, Vunjak-Novakovic G, Freed LE. In vitro differentiation of chick embryo bone marrow stromal cells into cartilaginous and bone-like tissues. J Orthop Res 1998;16(2):181-9.

36. Martin I, Shastri VP, Padera RF, Langer R, Vunjak-Novakovic G, Freed LE. Bone marrow stromal cell differentiation on porous polymer scaffolds. Trans Orthop Res Soc 1999;24:57.

37. Miura M, Gronthos S, Zhao M, Lu B, Fisher LW, Robey PG, et al. SHED: stem cells from human exfoliated deciduous teeth. Proc Natl Acad Sci U S A 2003;100(10):5807-12.

38. Nehrer S, Domayer S, Dorotka R, Schatz K, Bindreiter U, Kotz R. Three-year clinical outcome after chondrocyte transplantation using a hyaluronan matrix for cartilage repair. Eur J Radiol 2006;57(1):3-8.

39. Ohbayashi N, Shibayama M, Kurotaki Y, Imanishi M, Fujimori T, Itoh N, et al. FGF18 is required for normal cell proliferation and differentiation during osteogenesis and chondrogenesis. Genes Dev 2002;16(7):870-9.

40. Oshima Y, Watanabe N, Matsuda K, Takai S, Kawata M, Kubo T. Fate of transplanted bone-marrow-derived mesenchymal cells during osteochondral repair using transgenic rats to simulate autologous transplantation. Osteoarthritis Cartilage 2004;12(10):811-7.

41. Pittenger MF, Mackay AM, Beck SC, Jaiswal RK, Douglas R, Mosca JD, et al. Multilineage potential of adult human mesenchymal stem cells. Science 1999;284(5411):143-7.

42. Ponticiello MS, Schinagl RM, Kadiyala S, Barry FP. Gelatin-based resorbable sponge as a carrier matrix for human mesenchymal stem cells in cartilage regeneration therapy. J Biomed Mater Res 2000;52(2):246-55.

43. Selmi TA, Verdonk P, Chambat P, Dubrana F, Potel JF, Barnouin L, et al. Autologous chondrocyte implantation in a novel alginate-agarose hydrogel: Outcome at two years. J Bone Joint Surg Br

2008;90(5):597-604.

44. Shirasawa S, Sekiya I, Sakaguchi Y, Yagishita K, Ichinose S, Muneta T. In vitro chondrogenesis of human synovium-derived mesenchymal stem cells: optimal condition and comparison with bone marrow-derived cells. J Cell Biochem 2006;97(1):84-97.

45. Stevens MM, Marini RP, Martin I, Langer R, Prasad Shastri V. FGF-2 enhances TGF-beta1-induced periosteal chondrogenesis. J Orthop Res 2004;22(5):1114-9.

46. Takiguchi T, Kobayashi M, Suzuki R, Yamaguchi A, Isatsu K, Nishihara T, et al. Recombinant human bone morphogenetic protein-2 stimulates osteoblast differentiation and suppresses matrix metalloproteinase-1 production in human bone cells isolated from mandibulae. J Periodontal Res 1998;33(8):476-85.

47. Tsutsumi S, Shimazu A, Miyazaki K, Pan H, Koike C, Yoshida E, et al. Retention of multilineage differentiation potential of mesenchymal cells during proliferation in response to FGF. Biochem Biophys Res Commun 2001;288(2):413-9.

48. Vunjak-Novakovic G, Meinel L, Altman G, Kaplan D. Bioreactor cultivation of osteochondral grafts. Orthod Craniofac Res 2005;8(3):209-18.

49. Vunjak-Novakovic G, Obradovic B, Martin I, Bursac PM, Langer R, Freed LE. Dynamic cell seeding of polymer scaffolds for cartilage tissue engineering. Biotechnol Prog 1998;14(2):193-202.

50. Weissman IL. Translating stem and progenitor cell biology to the clinic: barriers and opportunities. Science 2000;287(5457):1442-6.

51. Wendt D, Jakob M, Martin I. Bioreactor-based engineering of osteochondral grafts: from model systems to tissue manufacturing. J Biosci Bioeng 2005;100(5):489-94.

"Science may set limits to knowledge, but should not set limits to imagination"

(Bertrand Russell)

Chapter 3.

The Current Status of Biomechanical Evaluation of the Hyaline Cartilage

Milan Handl, Milan Držík, Ferdinand Varga

Take Home Message

Studies have shown that impact-based testing have the feasibility, good replicability and overall reliability of the dynamic tests, even for such a mechanically complicated material like articular cartilage. This indicates promising possibilities for more comprehensive future studies of hyaline cartilage mechanical properties.

Introduction

Hyaline cartilage is an original congenital tissue, which when damaged is practically impossible to either fully restore or substitute with another tissue of similar quality. Nowadays there is frequently the demand for such an autogenous or artificial tissue for cartilage repair, which raises the question of how to compare the properties of both the original and substitute materials. Among other things, biomechanical testing provides a relatively exact and relevant method which can be used for this purpose. Of course, the various testing methods would need to be standardized so that they could be compared worldwide. This was also the reason why the authors decided to add this chapter: it presents another way of testing and evaluating hyaline cartilage biomechanics and its unique composition.

Joint function

The synovial joint, as e.g. in the knee needs to coordinate multiple connective tissues in order to function correctly. Hyaline cartilage covers the subchondral bone and thus provides a lubricated and nearly frictionless weight-bearing surface, protecting the joint's smooth function. Hyaline cartilage ensures good tissue integrity until 70 or 80 years of age even when the joint is functioning under high loads.

The knees are exposed to 5 to 10 times body weight forces during life activity, which is caused by the interaction between the highly viscous synovial fluid and the hyaline cartilage matrix. In normal joint loading, synovial fluid circulates and produces a weeping effect at the cartilage surface. The dynamic compression of the cartilage matrix provides movement of nutrients into the joint as well as into the hyaline cartilage via synovial fluid.

Cartilage structure and function

The hyaline cartilage in the synovial joints is formed by four distinct adherent zones. This structure prevents cartilage damage, which can be caused by load, tensile stress, injury etc. The four zones are the superficial tangential, the intermediate transitional, the deep radial and the calcified cartilage, the latter being at the junction with the subchondral bone. These zones are composed of 95 % extracellular matrix and 5 % chondrocytes as the exclusive cellular substance. They respond to mechanical and hydrostatic pressure changes. The extracellular matrix is composed of 75 % water, 20 % collagen (mostly Type II, also types IX and XI), 5 % proteoglycans and less than 1 % proteins (enzymes, lipids, growth factors etc).

Each of the cartilage zones has its special role. The tangential zone, composed of densely located collagen fibrils with parallel orientation, protects the cartilage surface from shear. The structure of the intermediate zone is formed by smaller and more spherical chondrocytes and obliquely oriented collagen fibrils. This zone protects the cartilage from shear and compressive forces. The deep zone is formed by the largest chondrocytes and its collagen fibrils are oriented perpendicularly. The function of this zone is to resist compressive forces. The zone of calcified cartilage is formed by the tidemark of calcified subchondral bone and superficially attached uncalcified cartilage. The function of this zone is dependent on the strength resistency of the cartilage.

Water is distributed through the extracellular matrix by mechanical compression and by the pressure gradient. When water moves through the extracellular molecular pores, high friction resistance is achieved. The solid, resilient cartilage is thus formed by the interactions between water, proteoglycans and collagen fibrills.

The cross-linked fibrillar structure of collagen is formed by three α chains in a triple helix. Collagen is responsible for the tensile stiffness, strength and stability of the hyaline cartilage. The mechanical behavior of the cartilage is determined by the diameter and orientation of these fibers, their density and the amount of collagen interfibrillar cross-links.
Chondrocytes produce glycosaminglycan aggregates and distribute them into the matrix in the form of proteoglycans. Proteoglycans bind or release water; by these means they are responsible for the compressive strength of the cartilage. Their concentration is lower in the superficial layer, with the highest being in the middle zones. Proteoglycan molecules form a network interacting with the collagen network, thus stabilizing the extracellular matrix.

Hyaline Cartilage Biomechanics

Hyaline cartilage consisting of both solid and liquid phases, is a viscoelastic tissue that is exposed to a wide spectrum of load conditions. Hyaline cartilage permeability is nonlinear, decreasing with increasing compression and vice versa. Thus, it shows time dependent behavior. Constant compressive stress causes tissue deformation until equilibrium is reached. In addition, stress-relaxation occurs with constant tissue deformation. This causes stress to rise to a maximum and then decrease over time until equilibrium is reached. Hyaline cartilage compression, shear and tensile forces can be described by two mechanisms: flow-dependent viscoelasticity and flow-independent viscoelasticity.
During short-duration cartilage compressive loading, fluid pressure provides support and the solid phase is protected in a type of stress shielding. The cartilage resists the compressive forces by the distribution of water. When the equilibrium state is achieved, tissue permeability and compressive stiffness are equal. Water moves through the cartilage under high pressure conditions. The cartilage compression yields a nonlinear effect, because porosity is reduced and the density of the negative charge contribution is increased. This mechanism disables the outflow of water from the hyaline cartilage matrix, which means respectively an increase in hydrodynamic forces and load-bearing capacity. Water from the matrix is delivered to the surface as a thin layer, so that the friction of the surfaces is minimized and their contact enables smooth gliding.

Mechanical properties, viscoelasticity

Strain is a relative measure of deformation. A stress-strain curve is simply the relationship of stress versus strain. When the linear stress-strain curve is proportional and the elastic deformation is fully recoverable, the relationship is known as Hook's law and Young's modulus of elasticity is defined as a slope of the curve.

When the elastic deformation range is defined as the limit after which the stress-strain ratio is no longer proportional, the stress-strain curve describes the material's toughness and thus characterizes its intrinsic properties.

Viscoelastic material shows the behavior of creep and stress relaxation. There are three principal differences in the mechanical response between viscoelastic and elastic material: (i) The mechanical response of viscoelastic material is time-dependant. A dependence on strain rate is present – the faster the deformation, the larger the stress required. Under constant loading, further strain develops – this phenomenon is called creep of the material. (ii) The loading and unloading curves do not coincide, but form a hysteresis loop. (iii) Permanent deformations may appear upon complete unloading, but delayed recovery of the material's original size and capabilities is also possible after some time. A further phenomenon worth mentioning is the phase angle, which characterizes the lag between the strain value's actual response and the instantly-applied stress. This feature, also typical for cartilage tissue, is characteristic for poroelastic materials and sometimes understood as a principal difference between poroelastic and viscoelastic substances[1,2].

Hyaline cartilage under a pure shear force can be described by flow-independent viscoelasticity. In this case, due to the collagen's organization in the middle zone, there is no fluid flow or tissue volume change that can occur. The collagen fibrils are stressed and provide resistance when shear forces are applied.

While the primary load-bearing purpose of the articular cartilage is to resist compressive loads, the material also provides tensile resistance. The intrinsic tensile properties of the collagen matrix can be tested by very slow loading conditions, whereby the stress-strain curve obtained represents the collagen matrix response to tensile force.

Physiological loading of hyaline cartilages

Water makes up the majority of native cartilage mass and plays the principal role in the tissue's ability to withstand large compressive forces. Solid cartilage structures are thus exposed to hydrostatic pressure. In diarthroidal joints this interstitial pressure ranges between 5 - 10 MPa and it is applied periodically during normal activities[3]. Considering loading dynamics, the acting force rises to a peak in approximately 100 ms during normal gait[4]. Corresponding typical loading rates in the order of 20 kN.s^{-1} and strain rates in the order of 5 s^{-1} occur in the tibio-femoral joint[5] . The loading time shortens to about 30 ms, and the loading rate increases to the order of 200 kN.s^{-1} during running[6] .

Examination of hyaline cartilage mechanical properties

As biological tissues are physically nonlinear materials, their dynamic properties (i.e. the viscoelastic storage and loss moduli) strongly depend on both the strain rate and the amplitude of the applied strain. An accurate experimental characterization of such material for its stress-strain response requires complete dynamic tests with varying rates of loading to obtain load-displacement curves.

In principle, the established methods for mechanical testing of cartilage tissue can be adapted from mechanical engineering standards, but often these tests do not give sufficient regard to the specifics of biological bearing elements as they are loaded *in vivo*. Specific features of the specimens, their small sizes and poorly-defined specimen geometries, their low material stiffness as well as their highly nonlinear and strain rate dependent nature have to be respected.

Quasistatic testing methods

Measurements are usually conducted via loading tests on universal testing machines (e.g. reference 7). There is a vast variety of commercially available testing devices allowing mechanical material testing in compression, tension, shear, torsion, flexion, fatigue, and examination of hardness or ductility. Conventional testing approaches involve constant loads, constant load-rates, and constant displacement-rates. As these modalities are quite ordinary in general material testing, they are also most common for evaluating cartilage tissue mechanical properties. Therefore, this kind of testing is primarily appropriate for low strain rate conditions.

Cyclic loading

In quasi-static testing there is an assumption that the material continually adjusts to applied pressure, which is not the case with dynamic testing, where changes are too fast to adapt to. In order to extend the possibilities of biological material testing, several measuring procedures based on cyclic loading have been proposed[8]. Due to the impossibility of avoiding fluid escape from the solid matrix after each cycle of compression loading, a considerable residual compression arises whereby the slope of the loading curve (material stiffness) increases cycle by cycle. Therefore, cartilage stiffness values in the initial cycles differ from those at the end of cycling interval.

Indentation techniques

Indentation techniques (e.g. references 9, 10) for compressive cartilage testing have gained major attention recently. A few hand-held indentation probes have been designed (e.g. reference 11). Indentation techniques generally examine a certain sample segment, which is surrounded by its natural environment (i.e. the surrounding cartilage tissue). A substantial benefit of indentation probes is that they can function arthroscopically. Although the technique is relatively simple in principle, the quantitative interpretation of experimental data is not always straightforward.

Ultrasonics

Ultrasonics is another testing method used to characterize the mechanical behavior of materials. Hattori et al.[12], Kukori et al.[13] and others evaluated echo duration and maximum magnitude in diagnostic frequency ultrasound examinations and found those specific for different grades of cartilage alteration as obtained in macroscopic classification. The exceptionally small-scale deformations and the relatively high-frequency loading applied by ultrasonic waves or nanoindentation are the characteristic features of this technique.

Alternative techniques

Studies employing other alternative approaches are less frequent. Berkenbilt et al.[14] applied small sinusoidal currents to the surface of hyaline cartilage to measure current-generated stress. Sachs et al.[15] used electromechanical spectroscopy to model the response of cartilage subjected to a periodic mechanical displacement applied to the articular surface. They found this nondestructive method was able to detect focal regions of cartilage degeneration. Dashefsky[16] utilized a microminiature pressure transducer to qualitatively assess chondromalacia of the patellar facet under arthroscopic control.

Impact testing

In order to better understand the behavior of the material as close as possible to *in vivo* conditions, several attempts have been made both to stimulate and measure the impact loading stress state[17,18]. The most common setup for these experiments is that the specimen placed on an anvil is struck by the free-falling mass of a guided impactor. As the early measurement methods in the drop-tower design could not estimate the descending part of the loading curve, attempts to evaluate the energy dissipation and also determine ultimate strength were hindered. Critical mechanical characteristics such as maximum dynamic modulus, maximum stiffness, stress and strain have been evaluated.

Pendulum-like impact testing system

In addition to high strain rates at loading, the drawback of dropped-weight testing is the impossibility of recording the unloading phase of the impact process. In an effort to avoid this limitation an instrumented pendulum-based test apparatus has been developed. In such testing the pendulum head strikes the specimen, which is positioned perpendicularly to its motion in a horizontal direction (Figs. 1 and 2). In contrast to the vertical drop-weight, the concept of the pendulum-based testing principle can provide important information about the energy conditions during the impact process.

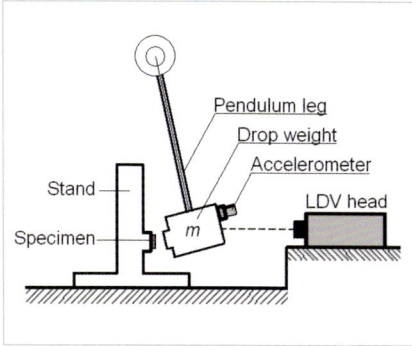

Figure 1: Set up of pendulum-like impact testing.

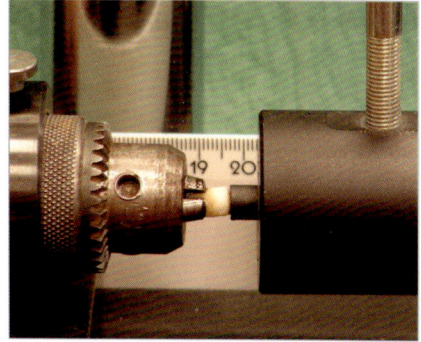

Figure 2: Cartilage sample in the testing device.

A pendulum-like apparatus setup permits the tracking of material response to a single impact, which can be adjusted to parameters approaching the physiological conditions of joint cartilage loading. The acting forces as well as stresses and actual sample deformations are evaluated from the processed piezoaccelerometer signals. The relationship of acting force or stress vs. deformation is then expressed by a loading diagram. Fig. 3 shows the typical force-displacement dependence of one of the native hyaline cartilage specimens under impact test by a pendulum type apparatus.

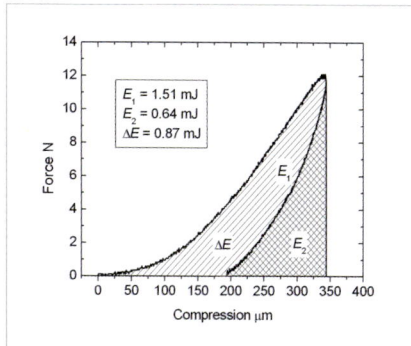

Figure 3: Experimentally achieved loading diagram illustrating impact energy balance. Total stored energy of impact denoted E_1 and restituted energy E_2. Their difference - area of hysteresis - is represented by the dissipated energy ΔE.

Biomechanical characteristics of hyaline cartilage

The variables such as Young's modulus of elasticity, the shear modulus, Poisson's ratio etc. may appear nonsatisfactory for a complex description of nonlinear poroelastic structures of interest. The entire loading diagram or instant quantities under defined load can serve for this purpose.

Stiffness is commonly characterized by the slope of the linear region of a force-deformation curve. Consequently, the stress-strain relationship is defined by a modulus of elasticity. As seen also from Fig. 3, there is no linear material behavior, so the tangent modulus has to be defined. For example, the statistical value of the stiffness at failure in the group of 18 native hyaline articular cartilage specimens that we tested was $(37.32 \pm 4.04) \cdot 10^3$ Nm^{-1}.

Values of the elasticity modulus in uniaxial confined compression have been reported in the range of 2-10 MPa[19,20]. Human knee cartilage was reported to possess a compressive modulus ranging from 1 MPa to 19,5 MPa depending on the sample's harvesting location (femur, tibia, patella)[17,18,21]. Stiffness (Young's modulus) reduction with cartilage degeneration, revealed in macroscopic as well as histological classification, was also reported in humans[22].

The dissipated energy is another considerable variable in evaluating native cartilage status or quality. The mechanical energy lost within the process of deformation - dissipated energy ΔE - can be evaluated as the difference between the kinetic energy of the striking body at the very beginning ($E1$) and very end ($E2$) of the deformation process. This is graphically represented by the area under the whole loading curve (ΔE) - the hysteresis loop (see Fig. 3 and 4).

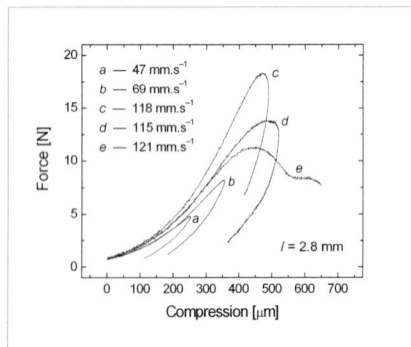

Figure 4: Force-compression loading curves of a single hyaline joint cartilage sample - consequent measurements a to e. Initial impact velocities v_1 are denoted for each measurement. Uncompressed sample thickness l = 2.8 mm.

Besides studying complete compressive loading curves, it is often also necessary to determine the compressive strength value. To obtain data for this ultimate value, the impact energy can be increased step-by-step up to apparent tissue failure. In contrast to prevailingly linear elastic and brittle materials, the failure limit of living tissue is not so strongly defined. Fig. 4 illustrates the example of hyaline cartilage blunt impact tests. The force-displacement graph of the intact cartilage (a, b, c) shows the successive increase in hysteresis with increasing impact velocity. Further, at approximately constant impact velocity, gradual degradation of tested material can be observed (c, d, e). The area of the hysteresis loop increases at the expense of plastic deformation, resulting in large residual deformation and overall cartilage material deterioration. The material is then damaged to the extent that the deformation is non-reversible, even after a long recovery period. This failure criterion was also similarly defined by e.g Repo and Finlay, and Kerin et al.[17,18]. These authors suggested that a decrease in the graph's gradient and a widening of the hysteresis curve indicates a region where irreversible damage and general failure occur. Thus, the dynamic loading curves recorded by the pendulum-like impact testing machine can reliably identify even the ultimate compressive strength. For impact loading, the accepted critical stress value causing chondrocyte death and ruptures in the extracellular matrix is $\sigma_{CR} = 15 - 20$ MPa[17,21,23]. Recently measured ultimate stress values causing irreversible damage of hyaline cartilage in impact testing range from $\sigma_{CR} = 16$ to 237 MPa, depending on the impact energy and strain-rate applied[24, 25] or $\sigma_{CR} = 11.32 \pm 2.32$ MPa at the corresponding strains $\varepsilon = 0.28 \pm 0.08$ as was demonstrated in our experiments by pendulum-like impact testing. Thus the principles of biomechanical properties of hyaline cartilage were compared to other sources from the literature[26].

Conclusions

The results obtained using impact-based testing have shown the feasibility, good replicability and overall reliability of the dynamic tests, even for such a mechanically complicated material. This indicates promising possibilities for more comprehensive future studies of hyaline cartilage mechanical properties.

References

1. Mow VC; Huiskes R (eds), Basic orthopaedic biomechanics and mechano-biology. Part 5, Lippincott Williams & Wilkins, 2005, 181-285
2. McCutchen CW, Cartilage is poroelastic, not viscoelastic (including an exact theorem about strain-energy and viscous loss, and an order of magnitude relation for equilibration time), Journal of Biomechanics, 1982, 15(4):325–327
3. Mow VC; Ratclife A; Poole AR, Cartilage and diarthrodial joints as paradigms for hierarchical materials and structures, Biomaterials, 1992, 13(2):67– 97
4. Bergmann G; Deuretzbacher G; Heller M; Graichen F; Rohlmann A; Strauss J; Duda GN, Hip contact forces and gait patterns from routine activities, Journal of Biomechanics, 2001, 34(7):859–871
5. Burgin LV; Aspden RM, A drop tower for controlled impact testing of bio¬logical tissues, Medical Engineering & Physics, 2007, 29(4):525–530
6. Aspden RM; Jeffrey JE; Burgin LV, Impact loading: physiological or patho¬logical?, Osteoarthritis and Cartilage, 2002, 10(7):588–589
7. Grellmann W; Berghaus A; Haberland EJ; Jamali Y; Holweg K; Reincke K; Bierogel C, Determination of strength and deformation behavior of human carti¬lage for the definition of significant parameters, Journal of Biomedical Materials Research part A, 2006, 78A(1):168–174
8. Barker MK; Seedhom BB, Articular cartilage deformation under physiological cyclic loading - apparatus and measurement technique, Journal of Biome¬chanics, 1997, 30(4):377–381
9. Bae WC; Temple MA; Amiel D; Coutts RD; Niederauer GG; Sah RL, Inden¬tation testing of human cartilage - Sensitivity to articular surface degeneration, Arthritis and Rheumatism, 2003, 48(12):3382–3394
10. Korhonen RK; Saarakkala S; Toyras J; Laasanen MS; Kiviranta K; Ju¬rvelin JS, Experimental and numerical validation for the novel configuration of an arthroscopic indentation instrument, Physics in Medicine and Biol¬ogy, 2003, 48(11):1565–1576

11. Lyyra T; Jurvelin J; Pitkanen P; Vaatainen U; Kiviranta I, Indentation instrument for the measurement of cartilage stiffness under arthroscopic control, Medical Engineering & Physics, 1995, 17(5):395–399

12. Hattori K; Mori K; Habata T; Takakura Y; Ikeuchi K, Measurement of the mechanical condition of articular cartilage with an ultrasonic probe: quanti¬tative evaluation using wavelet transformation, Clinical Biomechanics, 2003, 18(6):553–557

13. Kuroki H; Nakagawa Y; Mori K; Kobayashi M; Yasura K; Okamoto Y; Suzuki T; Nishitani K; Nakamura T, Ultrasound properties of articular cartilage in the tibio-femoral joint in knee osteoarthritis: relation to clinical assessment (Interna¬tional Cartilage Repair Society grade), Arthritis Research & Therapy, 2008, 10(4)

14. Berkenblit SI; Frank EH; Salant EP; Grodzinsky AJ, Nondestructive de¬tection of cartilage degeneration using electromechanical surface spectroscopy, Journal of Biomechanical Engineering - Transactions of the ASME, 1994, 116(4):384–392

15. Sachs JR; Grodzinsky AJ, Electromechanical spectroscopy of cartilage using a surface probe with applied mechanical displacement, Journal of Biome¬chanics, 1995, 28(8):963–976

16. Dashefsky JH, Arthroscopic measurement of chondromalacia of patella cartilage using a microminiature pressure transducer, Arthroscopy, 1987, 3:80–85

17. Repo RU; Finlay JB, Survival of articular-cartilage after controlled im¬pact, Journal of Bone and Joint Surgery - American volume, 1977, 59(8):1068–1076

18. Kerin AJ; Wisnom MR; Adams MA, The compressive strength of ar¬ticular cartilage, Proceedings of the Institution of Mechani¬cal Engineers Part H - Journal of Engineering in Medicine, 1998, 212(H4):273–280

19. Kempson GE, Mechanical properties of articular-cartilage, Journal of Physiology - London, 1972, 223(1):P23

20. Athanasiou KA; Agarwal A; Dzida FJ, Comparative-study of the intrin¬sic mechanical - properties of the human acetabular and femoral-head cartilage, Journal of Orthopaedic Research, 1994, 12(3):340–349

21. Varga F; Držík M; Handl M; Chlpík J; Kos P; Filová E; Rampichová M; Trč T;
Amler E, Biomechanical characterization of cartilages by a novel approach of blunt impact testing, Physiological Research, 2007, 56 (Suppl. 1): S61–S68

22. Kleemann RU; Krocker D; Cedraro A; Tuischer J; Duda GN, Altered carti¬lage mechanics and histology in knee osteoarthritis: relation to clinical assessment (ICRS Grade), Osteoarthritis and Cartilage, 2005, 13(11):958–963

23. Garcia JJ; Altiero NJ; Haut RC, An approach for the stress analysis of trans¬versely isotropic biphasic cartilage under impact load, Journal of Biome¬chanical Engineering - Transactions of the ASME, 1998, 120(5):608– 613

24. Burgin LV; Aspden RM, Impact testing to determine the mechanical proper¬ties of articular cartilage in isolation and on bone, Journal of Materials Science - Materials in Medicine, 2008, 19(2):703–711

25. Verteramo A; Seedhom BB, Effect of a single impact loading on the structure and mechanical properties of articular cartilage, Journal of Biomechan¬ics, 2007, 40(16):3580–3589

"The patient does not care about your science; what he wants to know is, can you cure him?"

(Martin H. Fischer)

CHAPTER 4.

POTENTIAL APPLICATIONS OF GENE THERAPY AND STEM CELLS TO ENHANCE ARTICULAR CARTILAGE REPAIR

Henning Madry, Magali Cucchiarini

Take Home Message

Based on emerging experimental data, it appears that gene transfer techniques and stem cells have a great potential for articular cartilage repair. In the future, gene transfer might be most beneficial when used in conjunction with established cartilage repair techniques. For stem cells, more experimental and clinical research is needed to further elucidate their mechanisms of action.

Introduction

The delivery by gene transfer methods of an interleukin-1 receptor antagonist (IL-1Ra) to synovial cells in the metacarpophalangeal joints of patients affected by rheumatoid arthritis some years ago[1] raised great scientific and clinical interest. For the treatment of cartilage defects that result from trauma or osteoarthritis however, the use of such gene-based technologies was so far restricted to animal models. Still, significant progress has been made by applying genetically modified cells that overexpress growth factors genes or potent gene vectors carrying genes for growth or transcription factors to articular cartilage defects.

Similarly in the past few years, the first reports documenting single cases of cartilage repair using bone marrow-derived stem cells were met with great clinical attention. Despite the interest generated, these early reports however did not provide any insight into the mechanisms of differentiation of the transplanted cells towards a chondrocyte phenotype. Moreover, no data on the dose-effect relationships or optimal administration parameters were provided. Surprisingly, although the scientific basis of the use of stem cells is currently weak, a number of clinical trials have been started. Yet, the results reported so far are rather modest and inconsistent.

The purpose of this chapter is to indicate the possible advantages and limitations of the current gene delivery approaches for application to cartilage defects. We will also outline the scientific bases of using stem cells for articular cartilage repair, comment on experimental studies, and outline possible directions of clinical research for the future.

2. Basic considerations

2.1. Basic considerations for gene therapy approaches

The process of repair after treatment of a cartilage defect with cell-based techniques such as articular chondrocyte transplantation or marrow-stimulation techniques shares similarities with the chondrogenic process observed during embryogenesis. Growth factors like the bone morphogenetic proteins 2 and 7 (BMP-2, BMP-7), fibroblast growth factor 2 (FGF-2), the members of the transforming growth factor beta (TGF-b) superfamily including TGF-b1 and TGF-b2 and the insulin-like growth factor I (IGF-I) have been shown to support chondrogenesis. Application of such factors in the form of recombinant molecules is largely not workable due to the very short intraarticular half-life of many of these agents.

The concept of using gene transfer strategies therefore originates from the theoretical possibility of transferring the genes for these factors to the repair tissue itself, resulting in a temporally and spatially optimal delivery of the therapeutic factor. With this strategy, transcription factors such as SOX9 that have an intracellular mode of action and a direct involvement in chondrogenic pathways may also be overexpressed.

Rather than stimulating anabolic responses as emphasized above, another strategy may be to prevent the long-term degeneration of the repair tissue by inhibiting degenerative pathways. Although potential targets have been described such as IL-1, no experimental data have been provided so far for the treatment of articular cartilage defects.

Targets for gene transfer include cells that play a role in the formation of the cartilaginous repair tissue, such as uncommitted mesenchymal stem cells or more mature, differentiated articular chondrocytes.

2.2. Basic considerations for stem cell approaches

The potential use of stem cells for cell-based therapy purposes, in particular those derived from the bone marrow compartment relies on their well-known regenerative effects during the spontaneous repair of osteochondral defects or when marrow-stimulation techniques are employed. The blood clot that spontaneously forms during these processes has an enriched content of such cells.

Stem cells are potentially an attractive alternative to the use of chondrocytes (like in autologous chondrocyte transplantation), as they are relatively easy to isolate in a rather non-invasive manner from a number of different tissues (bone marrow, but also adipose tissue, muscle, periosteum, and synovium). They have a capacity for self-renewal and retain a potential to differentiate into various specialized tissues, among which the articular cartilage.

Chondrogenesis of bone marrow-derived stem cells can be induced over a time of several weeks in culture if the cells are[1] maintained in high-density aggregate culture in the presence of specific factors among which[2] TGF-b and[3] dexamethasone[2].

3. Gene therapy approaches for cartilage repair

3.1. Overview

Strategies to deliver gene sequences into articular cartilage defects include the intraarticular injection of a gene vehicle or of genetically modified cells and an arthrotomy with either transplantation of ex vivo genetically modified cells or the direct administration of gene vectors into the cartilage defect (Figure 1).

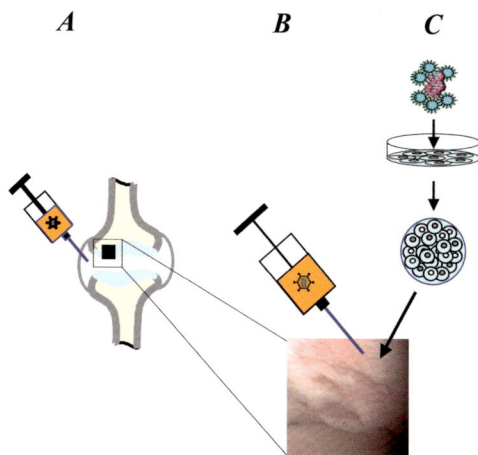

Figure 1: Strategies to deliver gene sequences into articular cartilage defects include (A) the intraarticular injection of a gene vehicle or of genetically modified cells and (B) the direct administration of gene vectors or (C) transplantation of ex vivo genetically modified cells into the cartilage defect, both via an arthrotomy.

3.2. Tools for gene therapy

Gene transfer is defined as being the introduction of foreign genes or gene sequences into somatic cells. Gene therapy is the treatment of diseases using gene transfer techniques. Gene transfer with nonviral vectors is called transfection whereas transfer via viral vectors is named transduction. As a result of the delivery, the genetic material enters the cell and is transferred to the nucleus where it either integrates into the host genome or remains extrachromosomal as episomal forms. In the latter case, expression of the transgene cassette is only transient. For applications such as overexpression of a growth factor, gene transfer into a sufficient number of target cells is necessary for the production of therapeutic amounts of the recombinant product. Techniques of gene transfer include physical, chemical, and viral transfer methods (Table 1).

Table1: Overview of currently mainly used gene transfer systems.

	Non-viral Systems	Viral Systems		
	Liposomes	Retroviral Vectors	Adenoviral Vectors	AAV Vectors
Advantages	• relatively high efficiency • low toxicity • transfection not cell cycle dependent • not immunogenic, repeatedly usable	• relatively high efficiency	• very high efficiency • transduction not cell cycle dependent	• very high efficiency • no induction of immun response • transfection not cell cycle dependent
Disadvantages	• efficiency is cell specific	• transduction cell cycle dependent • replication risk • unspecific intergration in genom	• induction of immune-response, therefore usability only once • replication risk	• helper-virus is necessary for production
Integration in Genom	• no	• yes	• no	• host dependent

Among the chemical methods, liposomes and non-liposomal lipid mixtures are popular components because of their safety and relatively high efficacy to transduce primary cells. Besides, viral vectors have raised attention due to the natural cell entry pathways of the viruses they are derived from. Vectors applied to date for gene therapy are mostly based on adenoviruses, retroviruses, and on the adeno-associated virus (AAV). Recombinant AAV (rAAV) vectors became a preferred viral transfer vehicle as a result of its low immunogenicity and low toxicity compared with adenoviruses, and because rAAV do not need cell division as a prerequisite for transgene expression in contrast to retroviruses, an advantage to target chondrocytes that generally do not divide. These properties of rAAV are due to the fact that all viral sequences are removed in the recombinant viral genome that is mostly maintained in the cells as episomes over extended periods of time. Most remarkably, transduction of a broad panel of primary cells (progenitors and committed cells) commonly occurs at very high efficiencies with this class of vectors compared with their counterparts.

3.3 Model systems in vitro

Gene transfer into articular chondrocytes and stem cells has been extensively studied in two-dimensional monolayer cultures. Genes can be introduced in articular chondrocytes using several nonviral methods[3] as well as adenoviral, retroviral, rAAV and lentiviral vectors[4]. Successful gene transfer in stem cells has been reported by several groups who employed nonviral vectors[5] or vehicles based on viruses such as adenoviruses[6], retroviruses[7], and AAV[8].

More relevant of a clinical situation, the use of three-dimensional systems has been recently advocated. These include the production of articular cartilage by tissue engineering approaches using transplantation of genetically manipulated articular chondrocytes in ex vivo model systems and the establishment of modified stem cells in three-dimensional conformations suited for chondrogenic differentiation. Concerning the application of modified articular chondrocytes, an interesting model is the transplantation of isolated and genetically modified articular chondrocytes onto articular cartilage explants, allowing for the creation of chimeric articular surfaces in vitro that are populated by genetically modified chondrocytes which form a new cartilaginous tissue. Overexpression of IGF-I, FGF-2, and BMP-7 vector in chondrocytes led to structural improvements of this new tissue[9-11].

Regarding stem cells, several groups demonstrated the feasibility of efficiently transducing progenitors by adenoviral[12], retroviral[13], and rAAV vectors[8] to place them in aggregate cultures where they could form cartilage-like cells by initiating chondrogenic differentiation. These studies served or may serve as a basis to establish gene transfer techniques for articular cartilage repair in vivo.

3.4. In vivo studies using genetically modified cells

Isolation of cells (articular chondrocytes, bone marrow-derived mesenchymal stem cells) prior to genetic modification is a prerequisite for transplantation purposes. After modification of these cells with a gene of interest, transplantation can be performed into the cartilage defect. This step usually employs cells that are attached to or embedded in supportive matrices (e.g. alginate) for containment inside the defect.

A preliminary study was performed by Kang and coworkers who transduced chondrocytes with a retroviral vector and embedded them in a fibrin gel. The authors reported the presence of transgene expression for 4 weeks[14]. Since, many other studies have described the use of nonviral, adenoviral, retroviral, or rAAV vectors using therapeutic genes like BMP-2 and BMP-7, IGF-I, FGF-2, and TGF-b[4].

Significant improvement in articular cartilage repair was noted in animal models depending on the gene applied. Most of these evaluations were performed in a rabbit model that is often used to screen genes of possible importance in the processes of cartilage repair. Hidaka and co-workers were the first to use a large animal model (horse) for ex vivo gene therapy approaches[15]. Allogeneic chondrocytes were transduced by an adenoviral vector carrying BMP-7 and next implanted into articular cartilage defects via arthroscopy. Although no structural difference was seen between the groups after 8 months, this was the first report including the biomechanical testing of repair tissue. Of note, several other large animal studies are currently ongoing.

Likewise, genetically modified bone marrow-derived mesenchymal stem cells have been used in animal studies for articular cartilage repair. Pagnotto et al. achieved improved cartilage repair in osteochondral defects when rAAV-TGF-b1-transduced hMSC were implanted[16].

In conclusion, transplantation of ex vivo modified cells has convincingly shown its potential to enhance articular cartilage repair. This strategy is particularly attractive for relevant applications in the future because all the technologies for the clinical preparation of articular chondrocytes are already in use for autologous chondrocyte transplantation. To envisage a clinical setting, a step of genetic modification ex vivo perhaps via nonviral vectors might be easily included. There are however currently no ongoing clinical studies known to the authors in this regard.

3.5. Direct application of gene transfer systems in vivo
Direct gene vector application to articular defects in vivo appeared difficult to achieve for a long time because many of the vector systems were not sufficiently effective to deliver directly genes into the articular cartilage. Specifically, non-viral, adenoviral, and retroviral vectors did not allow for a direct transgene expression in articular cartilage nor in the repair tissue formed after bone marrow stimulation techniques[4]. However, the use of rAAV vectors has significantly improved our capabilities of directly applying vectors to cartilage defects. rAAV are powerful tools to deliver genes either to chondral and osteochondral defects, mediating transgene expression for at least 4 months[17]. In these studies, transgene expression was also found in cells and tissues adjacent to the surgical procedure, such as the synovial membrane and quadriceps muscle. Application of therapeutic genes (FGF-2 alone or combined with SOX9) via rAAV vectors led to significant improvements of cartilage repair. The lack of adverse reactions over the period of observation in these experiments is an additional argument that may favor rAAV over more immunogenic adenoviral vectors. Nevertheless, in vivo studies using larger animals are still needed to corroborate the findings in the small rabbit model and it is noteworthy that no ongoing clinical trials have been initiated to date.

4. Stem cells

4.1. Overview
Stem cells have been delivered by intraarticular injection of isolated cells or in conjunction with supportive matrices. Direct intraarticular injection is the most simple approach, but their mechanism of action remains unclear. When stem cells are directly transplanted in an articular cartilage defect, their relative contribution to the defect repair with regard to other cells (e.g. from the synovial membrane or the underlying bone marrow) has not been elucidated.

4.2. Experimental studies using stem cells
There are only few experimental studies to date that have studied the treatment of articular cartilage defects with populations of mesenchymal stem cells. When chondral defects in the knee joints of minipigs were treated by direct intraarticular injection of stem cells suspended in hyaluronic acid, the cell-treated defects showed improved cartilage repair at 12 weeks compared with injections of saline or hyaluronic acid alone[18]. Im et al. have shown that implantation of rabbit mesenchymal stem cells from the bone marrow into osteochondral defects resulted in better histological scores and more intense immunohistochemical staining for type-II collagen after 14 weeks in vivo compared with the control[19]. Chang et al. used autologous uncultured bone marrow-derived mononuclear cells in a fibrin gel for transplantation in large full-thickness cartilage of the tibial plateau in rabbits[20]. At 12 weeks in vivo, defects treated with bone marrow-derived mononuclear cells had superior cartilage repair compared with defects treated with autologous uncultured peripheral blood-derived mononuclear cells in a fibrin gel, fibrin gel alone, or no treatment. To better characterize the use of mesenchymal stem cells, it might be worthwhile to perform studies evaluating dose-effect relationships and to directly compare this treatments with established techniques such as microfracture or application of articular chondrocytes.

4.3. Clinical studies using stem cells
The currently available clinical data are characterized by only a few case reports. In these studies, bone marrow aspirates (about 20 ml) were taken from the iliac crest of patients. Stem cells were next re-implanted in articular cartilage defects at relatively high cell concentrations of 107 cells/cm^2. In contrast to microfracture that yields a repair tissue based on a blood clot containing a mixture of cells including mesenchymal stem cells, the application of an enriched stem cell population might be more beneficial to support chondrogenesis in articular cartilage defects. In the published case reports, patients were 26-45 years old and the treated defects had sizes of about 3-5 cm^2[2,21-23]. The cells were applied in conjunction with collagen gels and a periosteal flap. Locations in the knee included defects in the condyles but also retropatellar and trochlear defects with kissing lesions. The resulting tissue was a often a thin repair cartilage identified as fibrocartilage. Calcification was observed in some cases, based on immunostaining that was positive for type-X collagen. For example, Wakitani et al. reported two cases of autologous bone marrow stromal cell transplantation for repair of full-thickness articular cartilage defects in human patellae[21]. One year after the first

and two years after the second transplantation, arthroscopy revealed a fibrocartilaginous defect repair. Another study by the same group reported improved arthroscopic and histological grading scores without clinical improvement for patients with knee osteoarthritis who underwent a high tibial osteotomy together with transplantation of mesenchymal stem cells embedded in a collagen gel and transplanted into cartilage defects in the medial femoral condyles covered with autologous periosteum, compared with patient receiving high tibial osteotomies alone without cells, without a collagen gel and without a periosteal flap[24].

5. Conclusions

Gene therapy and the use of stem cells still remain experimental strategies for articular cartilage repair, but significant scientific bases have been laid for their use.

5.1. Gene therapy
For gene therapy, a number of issues are still open. The use of gene therapy to treat nongenetic, nonlethal diseases such as cartilage defects (or osteoarthritis) requires that all possible safety concerns are adequately addressed.

A major technical limitation of the current protocols is the transient nature of transgene expression. Possible reasons for this phenomenon include the silencing of control elements regulating transgene expression, the loss of the gene vector, of the transduced cells, or both, and need to be better characterized.

When biomaterials are also used, it is critical that their presence does not impair the release of the therapeutic factor from the modified cells.

It is also unclear what the ideal growth factor will be in these approaches and whether a combination of several growth factors will be needed. Moreover, by closely regulating transgene expression, it might be possible to meet the sequence of events occurring during chondrogenesis.
Finally, it remains unlikely that gene therapy as a single procedure will replace clinical options to restore articular cartilage. As a matter of fact, gene transfer might be more beneficial when used in conjunction with surgical interventions such as marrow stimulation techniques.

5.2. Stem cells
On the basis of the available experimental evidence of the role of bone marrow-derived stem cells, it is difficult not to be optimistic about their potential for articular cartilage regeneration, but there are several points of interrogation that remain concerning their future use in clinical settings:

1. What is the optimal amount of cells per cartilage defect volume needed?

2. What is the fate of the cells once implanted? How long do they survive?

3. What is their influence on the repair of the lesion vis a vis local cells, such as cells from the bone marrow and synovial membrane?

4. What are the mechanisms of action involved in the repair processes? Does the occurrence of hypertrophy and type-X collagen expression sometimes observed in experimental studies play a role in vivo?

5. What are the possible interactions between the cells applied and the biomaterial that contain them in the defect?

6. Is the cartilaginous repair tissue hyaline or fibrocartilaginous?

7. What are the benefits of transplanting mesenchymal stem cells compared with articular chondrocytes?

In conclusion, it is likely that stem cells have a great potential and experimental data are emerging on their use for articular cartilage repair. However, little is known yet on their mechanisms of action and on the time course of application required to promote the healing of cartilage defects. Also, the clinical data available to support their use are still insufficient.

6. Outlook

Close interactions between scientists and clinicians will enable us to better address these questions in the future in order to develop accurate techniques that improve the healing of cartilage defects in patients. Yet, realizing the potential of gene transfer and stem cells requires a broad consensus among researchers and clinicians on the scientific evidence needed before experimental data can be translated into patients.

References

1. Evans CH, Robbins PD, Ghivizzani SC, et al. Gene transfer to human joints: progress toward a gene therapy of arthritis. Proc Natl Acad Sci U S A. 2005;102(24):8698-703.
2. Johnstone B, Hering TM, Caplan AI, Goldberg VM, Yoo JU. In vitro chondrogenesis of bone marrow-derived mesenchymal progenitor cells. Exp Cell Res. 1998;238(1):265-72.
3. Orth P, Weimer A, Kaul G, Kohn D, Cucchiarini M, Madry H. Analysis of novel nonviral gene transfer systems for gene delivery to cells of the musculoskeletal system. Mol Biotechnol. 2008;38(2):137-44.
4. Cucchiarini M, Madry H. Gene therapy for cartilage defects. J Gene Med. 2005;7(12):1495-1509.
5. Hoelters J, Ciccarella M, Drechsel M, et al. Nonviral genetic modification mediates effective transgene expression and functional RNA interference in human mesenchymal stem cells. J Gene Med. 2005;11:11.
6. Conget PA, Minguell JJ. Adenoviral-mediated gene transfer into ex vivo expanded human bone marrow mesenchymal progenitor cells. Exp Hematol. 2000;28(4):382-90.
7. Allay JA, Dennis JE, Haynesworth SE, et al. LacZ and interleukin-3 expression in vivo after retroviral transduction of marrow-derived human osteogenic mesenchymal progenitors. Hum Gene Ther. 1997;8(12):1417-27.
8. Ito H, Goater JJ, Tiyapatanaputi P, Rubery PT, O'Keefe RJ, Schwarz EM. Light-activated gene

transduction of recombinant adeno-associated virus in human mesenchymal stem cells. Gene Ther. 2004;11(1):34-41.

9. Madry H, Zurakowski D, Trippel SB. Overexpression of human insulin-like growth factor-I promotes new tissue formation in an ex vivo model of articular chondrocyte transplantation. Gene Ther. 2001;8(19):1443-9.

10. Madry H, Emkey G, Zurakowski D, Trippel SB. Overexpression of human fibroblast growth factor 2 stimulates cell proliferation in an ex vivo model of articular chondrocyte transplantation. J Gene Med. 2004;6(2):238-45.

11. Hidaka C, Quitoriano M, Warren RF, Crystal RG. Enhanced matrix synthesis and in vitro formation of cartilage-like tissue by genetically modified chondrocytes expressing BMP-7. J Orthop Res. 2001;19(5):751-8.

12. Kawamura K, Chu CR, Sobajima S, et al. Adenoviral-mediated transfer of TGF-beta1 but not IGF-1 induces chondrogenic differentiation of human mesenchymal stem cells in pellet cultures. Exp Hematol. 2005;33(8):865-72.

13. Lee K, Majumdar MK, Buyaner D, Hendricks JK, Pittenger MF, Mosca JD. Human mesenchymal stem cells maintain transgene expression during expansion and differentiation. Mol Ther. 2001;3(6):857-66.

14. Kang R, Marui T, Ghivizzani SC, et al. Ex vivo gene transfer to chondrocytes in full-thickness articular cartilage defects: a feasibility study. Osteoarthritis Cartilage. 1997;5(2):139-43.

15. Hidaka C, Goodrich LR, Chen CT, Warren RF, Crystal RG, Nixon AJ. Acceleration of cartilage repair by genetically modified chondrocytes over expressing bone morphogenetic protein-7. J Orthop Res. 2003;21(4):573-83.

16. Pagnotto MR, Wang Z, Karpie JC, Ferretti M, Xiao X, Chu CR. Adeno-associated viral gene transfer of transforming growth factor-beta1 to human mesenchymal stem cells improves cartilage repair. Gene Ther. 2007;14(10):804-13.

17. Cucchiarini M, Madry H, Ma C, et al. Improved tissue repair in articular cartilage defects in vivo by rAAV-mediated overexpression of human fibroblast growth factor 2. Mol Ther. 2005;12(2):229-238.

18. Lee KB, Hui JH, Song IC, Ardany L, Lee EH. Injectable mesenchymal stem cell therapy for large cartilage defects--a porcine model. Stem Cells. 2007;25(11):2964-71.

19. Im GI, Kim DY, Shin JH, Hyun CW, Cho WH. Repair of cartilage defect in the rabbit with cultured mesenchymal stem cells from bone marrow. J Bone Joint Surg Br. 2001;83(2):289-94.

20. Chang F, Ishii T, Yanai T, et al. Repair of large full-thickness articular cartilage defects by transplantation of autologous uncultured bone-marrow-derived mononuclear cells. J Orthop Res. 2008;26(1):18-26.

21. Wakitani S, Mitsuoka T, Nakamura N, Toritsuka Y, Nakamura Y, Horibe S. Autologous bone marrow stromal cell transplantation for repair of full-thickness articular cartilage defects in human patellae: two case reports. Cell Transplant. 2004;13(5):595-600.

22. Kuroda R, Ishida K, Matsumoto T, et al. Treatment of a full-thickness articular cartilage defect in the femoral condyle of an athlete with autologous bone-marrow stromal cells. Osteoarthritis Cartilage. 2007;15(2):226-31.

23. Wakitani S, Nawata M, Tensho K, Okabe T, Machida H, Ohgushi H. Repair of articular cartilage defects in the patello-femoral joint with autologous bone marrow mesenchymal cell transplantation: three case reports involving nine defects in five knees. J Tissue Eng Regen Med. 2007;1(1):74-9.

24. Wakitani S, Imoto K, Yamamoto T, Saito M, Murata N, Yoneda M. Human autologous culture expanded bone marrow mesenchymal cell transplantation for repair of cartilage defects in osteoarthritic knees. Osteoarthritis Cartilage. 2002;10(3):199-206.

*"The ordinary scientific man is strictly a senti-
mentalist. He is a sentimentalist in this essential
sense, that he is soaked and swept away by mere
associations"*

(Gilbert K. Chesterton)

Chapter 5.

Relevant Conditions in Animal Experiments for Clinical Challenge in Cartilage Tissue Engineering

Didier Mainard, Nathalie Presle, Pierre-Jean Francin,
Pascale Gegout, Pierre Gillet

Take Home Message

Animal experiments do commit the important ethical responsibility of researchers. The animal studies as a base for future clinical studies demand a well prepared study design, enough the follow up and the criteria for analysis should be also attentively selected and detailed.

Introduction

Cartilage is a complex tissue with a very important biomechanical function closely related to its biochemical structure. Cartilage lesions are among the most frequent injuries in orthopaedic practice and lead to the loss of the articular function and pain. Tissue engineering could offer new treatment opportunities for repair with possibly the replacement of a whole defect by a tissue-engineered construct. Since the original paper of William Hunter published in 1743, increasing insights on cartilage biology have been provided. Nevertheless, only few successful clinical and surgical applications arose from the many experimental studies obtained in animals and many questions remain to be clarified. We don't know for instance why cartilage displays limited regenerative capacity or why the progression of cartilage injuries occurs all over the time without any ways to prevent it. Consequently, no suitable healing or repair with optimal histological, biological and biomechanical properties for the newly synthesized cartilage tissue is not yet available. Only further basic investigations on cartilage biology will provide new advances on the complex molecular mechanisms underlying the repair of this articular tissue.

Animal models are powerful tools for studying elements of the cartilage repair process in great detail. They can be used to evaluate tissue-engineering techniques for the reconstruction of damaged human cartilage and to develop therefore new clinical approaches. However, many questions remain to be answered before a tissue-engineered cartilage is available for clinical implementation. These questions are related to the kind of the tissue repair and the clinical outcome. The goal to be reached may be either an early relief of clinical symptoms with the recovery of joint function, or a prevention of cartilage degeneration leading later to osteoarthritis or both. In fact, building a real hyaline cartilage is probably not necessary to achieve the early clinical goal but is required if the aim to the long term is to prevent the development of secondary osteoarthritis.

As experiments in animal models are the key steps before transposition of basic findings to the orthopaedic practice, the current review will discuss their benefits and their limitations with regard to the aim of the studies and the hypothesis to be tested, and will point out the parameters which are relevant for clinical applications[14].

Animal experiments

The objective for cartilage engineering is to produce articular tissue for functionnal restoration of a joint surface that appears anatomically, histologically, biologically, and mechanically close to the original one. The newly synthesized tissue should be also well integrated with the surrounding cartilage and the underlying bone. Preclinical models have been developed in order to restrict animal studies, including in vitro culture of human or animal cells and explants. Indeed all efforts to replace reduce and refine experiments must be undertaken according to the 3Rs concept as defined by Russel and Burch in 1959[10]. The simple in vitro systems provide valuable tools to determine an optimal cell type, the source of the cells, the need to use growth factor(s) and the type of scaffold that can be used for stimulation of differentiation of cells into tissues with optimal phenotypes[14]. Nevertheless, many in vitro strategies that appeared to be promising provided disappointing results when translated to whole animals. The complexity of biological systems cannot be fully appreciated by in vitro studies, more especially for cartilage which is in the vicinity of various secreting tissues such as the synovium. These initial testings have therefore to be completed by experimental investigations. Animal models are in fact unavoidable to study the interaction between the environment and the engineered cartilage tissue, and to identify conditions which can stimulate cartilage repair and which can protect the newly synthesized tissue from further destruction induced by the surrounding joint tissues[5]. In addition, animal models can mimic clinical conditions and underline therefore the therapeutic applicability of the approach for cartilage repair. While no animal model permits direct application to humans, each is capable of yielding principles on which decisions can be made that might eventually translate into a human application. Clearly, the use of animal models has and will continue to play a significant role in the progress of the orthopaedic practice, and it is the duty of scientists to explain this important point to the non scientist population. Of course, as for clinical investigations, experimental studies in animal have to be conducted according to the ethical rules. In many countries, institutional use and care animal committees have now been established and approval of these committees is compulsory before beginning any animal study[10]. At international level, an European convention has therefore described the limitations and the conditions for the protection of vertebrate animals used for experimental and other scientific purposes and recalled the moral obligation of researchers in animal experiments[1].

Study design

Each animal model has specific advantages and disadvantages. The key issue in the selection of a suitable animal model is to match the model to the question being investigated and the hypothesis to be tested[4,5]. Consequently, a study design is essential to draw scientific conclusions. Studies on tissue bioengineering require preliminary data on the feasibility according to the engineering principles which can need a theoretical adjustment. The in vitro study follows this preliminary step and aims to select the cell type and the scaffold that can be used to obtain the optimal engineered cartilage tissue with the most effective interactions between cells and scaffold. The therapeutic applicability is thereafter examined in animal models. A first in vivo study uses most often heterotopic chondrogenesis model to establish in animal the potential chondrogenic properties of the tissue engineered construct. The last experimental step before a potential clinical application uses articular defect models which need larger animals with mid and long term follow up. These preclinical models aim to determine the quality of the cartilage repair directly in the joint, and have to be as close as possible of the clinical conditions.

It is worth noting that changes in the initial concept or in the study design, or a comeback to in vitro examinations can occur at each step even at the last one. In addition, one has to keep in mind the constraints for clinical applications and for industrial manufacture all along the investigations[5].

Heterotopic chondrogenesis animal models

This initial in vivo experiment aims at identifying all the parameters operating at the prospective implantation site[14]. For example a subcutaneous air pouch is created at the dorsal aspect of the back to form an in vivo reactor in which the construct may be implanted. The biological responses and the biocompatibility, as well as the ability to produce chondrogenic tissue are therefore examined during the course of the study[14]. Small animals as rodents (mice, rats) may be useful in the heterotopic chondrogenesis models but compromised nude mice are the most suitable. This easy to use model bridges the gap between the in vitro study and the articular defect models. The data obtained from the pilot study will be determinant for the next step, i.e. examinations of the engineering cartilage tissue in an articular defect animal model or further in vitro experiments.

Articular defect animal models

Many items have to be taken into account and kept in mind for critical evaluation and lecture about animal experiments on cartilage repair: the type, the size and the site of the lesion, the species, the age of the animal, the post-operative conditions, the follow-up, the criteria and the methods used for analysis, and the control groups[4]. Each animal model has specific advantages and disadvantages.

Type of lesion
As different clinical situations with different surgical care objectives may exist, two experimental models have been developed according to the damage tissues: a partial thickness cartilage defect and a full thickness cartilage defect[6,7,11,12]. The partial thickness cartilage defect affects a single tissue and is characterized by a transient and ineffective chondrocyte proliferation and a matrix synthesis near the margins, but without real healing mechanisms. By contrast, the lesion reaches the subchondral bone in the full thickness cartilage defect and induce an inflammatory response with exposure of the bone marrow and a subsequent recruitment of subchondral MSC which are able to repair spontaneously the lesion with fibrocartilagenous tissue. For each experimental model, the cartilage defect has to be reproducible in size and volume.

The acute or chronic feature of the lesion is another important point to be emphasized[14]. Animal models exhibit fresh and cartilage defect without joint trauma. By contrast, in the clinical situation, there is most often a long time between the trauma and the surgical treatment, and cartilage lesion has to be considered as a chronic damage with loss of joint homeostasis, inflammation, synovitis, effusion…As any changes in the joint homeostasis may disrupt cartilage repair, the experimental models can not match really with the clinical situation.

Some studies with cartilage defect animal models did not describe the method used to make the lesion. Various methods are now available including drilling, scalpel, curette or special dedicated device. They may influence the quality of the lesion and more especially the reproducibility of the defect, as well as the stresses and the strains on the surrounding cartilage. The washing of the joint is also important to report as suppression of mediators produced by other articular tissues may improve cartilage repair. Consequently, standardization of experimental conditions are required for suitable conclusions and comparisons.

Size of lesion

As large cartilage defects cannot be spontaneously repaired, it is necessary to define a critical size of lesion for every animal species used. Lesion sizes are often very different from a study to another one, even for the same species, preventing any comparison of the various findings. Further investigations are therefore required to evaluate the effect of the lesion size on the repair process and so to standardize this parameter in the different animal models.

The size is generally larger in large animals and smaller in small animals, but more importantly is the ratio between the damaged surface and the whole joint articular surface. For the same surface, this parameter may be very different in a small or a large animal, and a too large surface may be a bias for studying cartilage healing. The ratio length on width of the lesion is another parameter to be considered to avoid bias in the understanding of mechanisms underlying cartilage repair. In fact, surface and depth are determinant for the volume of the defect. The size of the chondrocytes and their ability to synthetize the extracellular matrix remain unchanged whatever the species, but the number of cells vary according to the species. A defect in cartilage may suppress a high number of cells in some species preventing spontaneous repair of the articular tissue. Consequently, the volume of the experimental lesion should take into account the number of chondrocytes in the cartilage of the animal used for the study[4].

The depth of the defect is also important to determine if the lesion is chondral or osteochondral. Deep lesions reaching the subchondral bone may induce some deleterious changes including the formation of a large cavity a collapse of the surrounding bone and cartilage which may interfere with mechanisms of cartilage healing.

In conclusion, the size, the volume and the depth of the lesion should be more standardized in all studies for each species according to the aims of the investigations.

Site of lesion

Many different locations in the joints are proposed by various authors as lesion knee : the medial or lateral femoral condyle, the medial or lateral tibial plateau, the patella, and the patella grove.

One more time, it is difficult to compare results of healing in different sites, especially between sites in weight and non-weight bearing area. It is now well established that biomechanical loading affects chondrocyte metabolism, indicating that cartilage repair may be strongly changed according to the location of the defect[8]. The locomotion of the species may also affect the healing process. As two third of the cartilage lesions in human are located in medial condyle, experimental lesions in large animal models should be always generated in weight bearing area of the medial femoral condyle[2].

Species

As previously explained, experimental studies for cartilage repair need small and large animals according to the stage of the investigations. Whatever the species used, animals have to come from a registered breeding establishment approved by the health authorities. In the literature, the choice of the animals ranges from mice to horses. Small animals such as mice, rats or rabbits are easy to handle and to store, and are cost efficient compared to larger animals.

Rabbits are the most commonly animals used for studies on cartilage repair. This choice is not however the most appropriate as cartilage healing in rabbits is often better than in other small animals and may be a little too favourable. That is why a comparative study between two different species may be advised.

Beside, studies in larger animals are required because their joints are closer to those found in human compared to joints of small animals, even if large animals are more difficult to handle, to operate and to store, and also more expensive. In addition, biomechanical stimuli and strain are more important in large than in small animals. Many species have been used in the literature: dogs, sheeps, pigs, goats, horses. ICRS recommends the goats for examining cartilage repair. Of course, many physiological and anatomical differences remain between large animals and humans about standing position, locomotion, weight bearing, range of motion…Moreover, there are intrinsic differences in articular structures between animals and humans[4]. That is why good findings in preclinical studies are prerequisite conditions before clinical applications, but not sufficient to be sure to have the same results in humans[5,14].

Other parameters

- Age of the animal

The age is a well-known factor which affects the healing process of cartilage and the response to the experimental treatment. Because spontaneous cartilage repair is better in immature than in skeletally mature animal, adult animals have to be chosen to be close to the clinical situation. For instance, the age of a rabbit must be over 4 months and over 6 to 8 weeks for a rat. It is also necessary to have homogeneous groups regarding the age of the animals. A variation of several months in some animals may represent several decades in humans.

- Weight of the animal

The weight of the animals of the experimental group must also be homogenous otherwise the biomechanical conditions will be not the same for all animals and that can modify the results from an animal to another. Biomechanical stimuli and strain are more important in large than in small animals.

- Gender of the animal

The influence of the gender of animals on results in cartilage repair is not clear. It seems preferable that the gender is the same for all the animals.

Statistical analysis

Of course, control groups and statistical analysis have to be considered as for human clinical trials. Sample size has to be in accordance with the expected results coming either from previous experiments or from the literature.

Post-operative conditions

It is not always easy to control post-operative conditions in animals but it may change the quality of healing. Total, partial or no weight bearing conditions, as well as walking and immobilization, influence the biomechanical stress on the cartilage and the lesion. Active or passive motion induced in some species also may also affect the quality of the repair. The post-operative conditions should be therefore be described in the study protocol and should be taken into account in the data analysis and in the discussion.

Follow up

Three to 4 time points should be provided together with a short mid and long term follow up. A short and mid term may be sufficient for a preliminary study in small animals, but a long term follow up over 6 months in larger animal should be compulsory before clinical application. A short term follow up under one month aims to study inflammatory and immunological responses while a mid term follow up from one to 3 months determines whether the tissue formed from the implanted construct is structurally and functionally relevant. The newly synthesized tissue must be therefore thoroughly characterized. Over 6 months of follow up one assesses the structural and the functional properties of the healing tissue in the long term, the potential development of a degenerative process over time, and the quality of the integration with the surrounding cartilage and the underlying bone. Time of follow up is different for each species. A couple of months are a long term for rats but a mid term for goats.

Results assessments

Results assessments need appropriate and well defined tissue sampling strategy (4). The choice of relevant parameters is a interdisciplinary decision according to the aims of the study in order to get reproducible, reliable and standardized means of evaluation. Quantitative or semi-quantitative scoring has to be prioritized to subjective scoring[14]. Pineda[15] and O'Driscoll[16] scorings are well recognized. They authorized reliable and good comparison and correlation between studies[15, 16]. Evaluation requires several observers blinded to group assessment. If needed, the surrounding tissues (synovium, subchondral bone), the synovial fluid and also local or regional lymph nodes and filtring organs may be examined. Except macroscopic appearance and histological analysis, many other criteria may be interesting for cartilage healing evaluation : SEM or MEB, immunohistochemistry, confocal laser microscopy, incorporation of radiolabelled precursor in the newly synthesized extracellular matrix. MRI which avoids sacrifices of the animals and permits longitudinal studies, may also provide informations on morphological and biochemical (spectrometry) parameters. High field MRI especially devoted to small animals (7 Teslas) or larger animals are now available, but clinical MRI are not allowed for large animal studies[9]. In small animals, the joint function may be quantitatively evaluated using telemetry[3]. Gait analysis or measurement of hind paw weight ratio as an index of joint pain by incapacitance can be performed as a clinical parameter to study the pain associated with the post chirurgical condition[13]. Finally, arthroscopy in large animals some devices as Artscan 1000 may give new findings on the biomechanical properties of cartilage.

Conclusion

Animal experiments based on relevant scientific criteria are strongly useful for cartilage tissue engineering. Because therapeutic approaches in patients with cartilage defect are based on the initial findings in experimental models, future researches in the most suitable animal model should be aimed at investigating and evaluating tissue repair in the best standardized conditions for the size, the type and the site of the lesion. The design of the study, the follow up and the criteria for analysis should be also attentively selected and detailed. Animal experiments do commit the ethical responsibility of researchers.

References:

1. European convention for the protection of vertebrate animals used for experimental and other scientific purposes. Council of Europe, ETS n° 123.
2. Hjelle K; Solheim E; Strand T; Muri R, Brittberg M, Articular cartilage defect in 1000 knee arthroscopies, Arthroscopy, 2002, 18 (7): 730-734.
3. Gegout-Pottie P; Philippe L; Simonin MA; Guingamp C; Gillet P; Netter P; Terlain B, Biotelemetry : an original approach to experimental models of inflammation,
Inflamm. Res., 1999, 48: 417-424.
4. Hunziker E, Biologic repair of articular cartilage, Clin. Orthop., 1999, 367: 135-146.
5. Hunziker E; Spector M; Libera J; Gertzman A; Woo S; Ratcliffe A; Lysaght M; Coury A; Kaplan D; Vunjac-Novakovic G, Translation from research to applications,
Tissue Engineering, 2006, 12 (12): 3341-3364.
6. Jackson DW; Lalor PA; Aberman HM; Simon TM, Spontaneous repair of full thickness defects of articular cartilage in a goat model, J. Bone Joint Surg., 2001, 83-A (10): 1591-1592.
7. Jansen EJ; Emans PJ; Van Rhijn LW; Bulstra SK; Kuijer R, Development of partial thickness articular cartilage injury in a rabbit model, Clin. Orthop., 2008, 466, 487-494.
8. Jung M; Breusch S; Daecke W; Gotterbarm T, The effect of defect localization on spontaneous repair of osteochondral defect in a Gottingen minipig model, Lab. Anim., 2009, 43 (2): 191-197.
9. Kangarlu A; Gahunia HK, Magnetic imaging characterization of osteochondral defect repair in a goat model at 8 T, Osteoarthritis Cartilage, 2006, 14, 52-62.
10. Kolar R, Animal experimentation. Sci. Eng. Ethics, 2006, 12 (1): 111-122.
11. Lahm A; Uhl M; Edlich M; Erggelet C; Haberstroh J; Kreuz PC, An experimental canine model for subchondral lesions of the knee joint, Knee, 2005, 12, 51-55.
12. Lu Y; Markel MD; Swain C; Kaplan LD, Development of partial thickness articular cartilage injury in an ovine model, J. Orthop. Res., 2006, 24, 1974-1982.

13. Pomonis JD; Boulet JM; Gottshall SL; Phillips S; Sellers R; Bunton T; Walker K, Development and pharmacological characterization of a rat model of osteoarthritis pain, Pain, 2005, 114 (3): 339-346.

14. Reinholz GG; Lu L; Saris DBF; Yaszemski MJ; O'Driscoll SW, Animal models for cartilage reconstruction, Biomaterials, 2004, 25, 1511-1521.

15. Pineda S; Pollack A; Stevenson S; Goldberg V; Caplan A, A semiquantitative scale for histologic grading of articular cartilage repair, Acta Anat (Basel), 1992, 143 (4): 335-340.

16. O'Driscoll SW; Marx RG; Beaton DE; Miura Y; Gallay SH; Fitzsimmons JS, Validation of a simple histological-histochemical cartilage scoring system, Tissue Eng. 2001, 7 (3): 313-320.

"Education is what survives when what has been learned has been forgotten"

(B. F. Skinner)

CHAPTER 6.

SUBCHONDRAL BONE: CURRENT CONCEPTS

James B. Richardson

Take Home Message

• *When both bone and cartilage are diseased then both need to be regenerated. Do not forget the cartilage-bone unit.*
• *Subchondral bone pathology is either generalized or localized can be dealt with in isolation.*
• *Generalized pathology is usually associated with instability or malalignment or meniscal loss. These underlying causes need to be addressed.*

Introduction

Subchondral bone is the life partner of cartilage. What affects one influences the other:
- Cartilage provides the low friction surface that disseminates shear and allows a joint to convert bending forces into axial loads sustained by the skeleton.
- Subchondral bone must be sufficiently flexible as if too stiff it becomes an anvil on which cartilage can be injured.

Causes of cartilage failure

Subchondral bone thickening as a cause of cartilage failure was proposed by Radin as a significant cause of cartilage loss[14]. This theory remains open to debate, but subchondral stiffening is in the author's opinion the substantial cause of osteoarthritis. Published knowledge in this field fails to explain how the normal homeostatic mechanisms fail to control this rise in stiffness.

Bone ingrowth into areas of healing cartilage defects is relatively common following microfracture, and may be seen in end-stage osteoarthritis as an 'internal osteophyte'. More widespread expansion of bone into cartilage was proposed by Hulth to account for cartilage thinning and osteoarthritis[8] but the prevalence of this method of joint failure is undefined.

The theoretical origin of cartilage failure will continue to be debated, but once the subchondral bone is diseased it is important that this is addressed as much as the overlying cartilage. In avascular necrosis, and less commonly in osteochondritis dissecans, the overlying cartilage is relatively healthy. Removing and grafting the underlying bone will not allow strong re-attachment of the overlying cartilage. This is important to recognize. When disease intervenes on the partnership of cartilage and bone, cartilage can grow and re-attach to bone, but if subchondral bone has to be replaced, the combined unit of bone and cartilage will need reconstruction.

High T2 signal on MRI

Acute high T2 signal on MRI following injury has a very different clinical correlation compared with a high signal seen in chronic situations. A significant observation in a study by Raynauld et al.[15] found a strong and independent association between the size of this signal and loss of cartilage volume. Cyst size also increased in association with cartilage loss, emphasizing the importance of subchondral bone pathology in osteoarthritis. Cysts were seen to follow areas of bone 'oedema-like signal' in another longitudinal study, and 87% of cysts had an adjacent area of abnormal cartilage[7].

Cyst formation

If low friction and wear are the primary functions of cartilage then protecting bone from high fluid pressures is the second contribution of this partnership. Cyst formation in osteoarthritis is relatively common and two main theories of causation are proposed. Bone absorption will follow exposure to high fluid pressures[22] and communication to the joint can be identified in some of these fluid-filled cysts. Other cysts are filled with fatty soft tissue and are thought to originate in the subchondral bone from spontaneous absorption. A macrophage infiltrate is commonly seen in enlarging cysts, and there is some evidence that these cells can differentiate into osteoclasts relatively easily[16].

The biomechanics of a cyst favour continued expansion. LaPlace's law states that 'the larger the vessel radius, the larger the wall tension required to withstand a given internal pressure'. As with blowing a party balloon, getting it started is the difficult bit!

Dickkopff

Dkk-1 is a hormone that acts high in the hierarchy of mesenchymal cell control, acting on WNT-signalling[12]. High levels are associated with cartilage formation, and low levels with bone formation, so it has the potential to control the switch between bone and cartilage formation. Our group has identified a non-union cell in atrophic non-unions for example that although senescent, secretes high levels of Dkk-1[4]. This might explain why bone is slow to form and cartilage appears in the non-union.

High levels of Dkk-1 are seen in the subchondral bone of patients with osteoarthritis and those with a tendency to osteoporosis have low levels, and this correlates with low prevalence of osteoarthritis. The 'Dkk-1 balance' may explain this spectrum that ranges between those with strong bone and arthritis, to those with osteoporosis but no arthritis. There could be therapeutic potential in controlling this balance.

Where does the pain originate?

Pain is thought of as a problem, but it has an essential function in protecting joint function. Loss of pain in the Charcot joint results in rapid destruction of the joint. Rapid onset of pain following injury is particularly useful and this is achieved by nerve fibres. Cartilage is devoid of these but subchondral bone has a rich supply which reaches to the subchondral plate.

Patients may have few symptoms while cartilage thins. Once bone is exposed then pain comes with activity. High friction transmits high local loads and local fractures occur in the cancellous bone. These fractures each heal with extra bone formation. Intense remodelling ensues. Bailey and co-workers have reported a 20-fold increase in remodelling and a 25% reduction in mineralization.

Loss of 'packing' on one side of the knee – the thinning of cartilage, loss of meniscus, and then loss of bone – leads to malalignment such that more weight is then transferred across the injured side of the joint. All these factors contribute to stiffening of the sub-chondral bone.

In other patients the malalignment follows other pathology or more commonly malunion. Personal experience is that shortening is more likely to lead to arthritis in the knee than malalignment, and indeed severe malalignment reduces activity levels and so indirectly protects against arthritis.

How does the theory translate to practice?

Subchondral bone pathology is either generalized or localized.
- Localized ones are cysts and osteochondral defects and can be dealt with in isolation.
- Generalized pathology is usually associated with instability or malalignment or meniscal loss. These underlying causes need to be addressed.

Where there is a combination of meniscectomy with ACL rupture then both me-niscal transplantation (AMT) and ACL repair are needed. Meniscal transplanta-tion in the presence of chondral loss had been contra-indicated but we reported success where AMT was combined with ACI[5]. In a group of 8 patients with bone-on-bone cartilage loss, success was achieved in 5 patients who have continued to have good function now out to 9 years of follow-up.

Osteotomy is designed to address malalignment and two good randomized tri-als confirm that new cartilage will form, but only if the subchondral bone has been exposed before the osteotomy is undertaken[2,18]. This is counter-intuitive, but confirms that although cartilage does not readily regenerate in the adult, it will repair with fibrocartilage once the wear has reached the level of the bone. In the study by Akizuki the effect of debridement was to improve the histologi-cal grade of repair, in the study by Schultz microfracture improved histology. In neither study was a clinical improvement seen but neither study included large numbers.

Osteotomy also causes a reduction in bone density through a stimulus to intense bone remodelling. Finsen found both the proximal tibia and distal femur lost around 10% in bone density following a proximal tibial closing osteotomy (Fin-sen, 1987). This osteopenia is commonly seen distal to any fracture in the lower limb. This remodelling must reduce the stiffness of the subchondral bone and may be a significant contribution to pain relief.

Fixation of the osteotomy as with fracture fixation has greatly improved with the development of more fixed angle devices. The Puddu technique has led the way with opening wedge osteotomy but some problems of instability have been reported[21]. A particular problem with the opening wedge is of fracture of the opposite cortex. I developed a tensegrity osteotomy where two bio-replaceable conical screws are used to open the wedge and these remain in compression with the plate in tension. The separation of tension and compression in different parts of the construct provide tensegrity.

Osteotomy of the femur is now rarely used for the management of early arthritis of the hip. Hip resurfacing is proving very effective at pain reduction and restores self-assed Harris hip scores to over 90 and Kaplan-Meir survival of a group of 800 patients with a minimum of 10 year follow-up is 94%[11]. I have combined ACI in the hip of 14 patients (unpublished) with bone grafting is these circumstances and found poor results where there is cyst formation in the hip.

When should high tibial osteotomy be advised? When is it better to proceed directly to unicompartmental knee replacement?

A randomised clinical trial in Hannover reports excellent or good results in 71% of 32 patients having osteotomy compared with 65% of 28 having unicompartmental knee replacement. Strangely the authors encourage use of the prosthesis[20]. The patient with early arthritis has to consider the life-time functional outcome. How will the two groups compare at 20 years after many have a total knee replacement? These answers will be difficult to obtain as they need long-term study.

Another development in osteotomy at the knee is the vertical cut or geometric osteotomy. I see four advantages to this development which I have used in proximal and distal femur, and in the proximal tibia. In all area it controls axial rotation, improves rigidity and stability, improves healing surface areas. In the high tibial osteotomy it also avoids displacing the patella distally which is important as by later stages there is a degree of osteoarthritis in the patello-femoral joint also.

Localised loss of bone in the absence of contributing factors will need more localised treatment. In the ankle a local osteochondral defect may heal well with simple cancellous bone grafting. Subchondral bone pathology dictates outcome in the ankle. In a study of 48 symptomatic patients, the 27 with subchondral necrosis or the 3 with extensive cysts had poorer outcome and persisting changes[10]. The Oscell cartilage service at Oswestry has a good experience of ACI in the ankle with a pre-operative Mazur ankle score of 54 maintained at 54 in 23 patients followed out to a maximum of 10 years[19].

In the knee a loose osteochondral fragment will not heal unless the intervening layer of cartilage is removed. Proteoglycans resist the vascular invasion necessary for bony union. Rigid fixation will aid healing.

Failure of cartilage repair

Excellent regenerate can follow a range of repair procedures in a joint but some fail and have persisting pain and local tenderness at 2 to 4 years. Technetium bone scan reveals a high level of activity in the late phase. MRI shows chronic bone oedema. Pain relief follows removal of this bone. These observations confirm the need to address all aspects when a cartilage defect is seen: alignment, stability and underlying bone inflammation.

Lateral integration of mature cartilage surfaces rarely occurs. The function of cartilage as a 'waterproofing layer' is lost and joint fluid under pressure reaches subchondral bone and leads to cyst formation. This problem can be addressed by the use of combined autologous chondrocyte implantation with mosaicplasty[17]. Chondrocytes in suspension will attach to freshly cut cartilage[24] and so provide good lateral integration between the grafted cartilage and the surrounding cartilage.

The second biological problem is of stress-induced apoptosis of chondrocytes. Techniques where high impact loads are applied to the graft during insertion result in apoptosis of the chondrocytes at the periphery of the graft. An interesting study found apoptosis more of an issue when the mosaic plug is slightly long for its drilled hole[13]. New cells will appear in these areas as apoptosis is a quiet method of cell turnover that does not induce inflammation. Equipment that minimizes this problem is expensive but probably necessary to get consistently good results.

The physical problems are difficult to overcome. Cartilage varies in thickness and so it is difficult to obtain grafts that match the treated site. Either cartilage or bone levels will therefore not match. Access to the tibial surface is difficult but has been overcome with angled techniques. The main problem is that if large areas need treatment then there is a lack of donor cartilage available. Again the combination of ACI and mosaicplasty is a help as the new plugs can be spaced out to cover a larger area.

Bone plugs

Carbon Fibre was widely used in the 1980's to treat chondral defects. Inadvertently the drill holes may have removed some underlying inflamed bone. Clinical benefits must have been convincing for such widespread use, and it was only with the presentation of carbon particles in the knee that it fell from favour. The mechanism of action is that the parallel bundles direct cells from deep in the subchondral bone to exit on the surface where they form well-attached pads of fibrocartilage. Mats Brittberg uses carbon fibre plugs as an effective option for revision cases.

Absorbable plugs

Considering the history of carbon fibre plugs I predict that an absorbable plug that works in the same manner will be widely useful. OBI produced a polycaprolactone with calcium sulphate plug on the basis of a deep layer that was stiff and a surface layer that is flexible. Surgeons report variable results and there are few reports to help identify the appropriate patients to select. Some report poor quality tissue in the deep part, and unpredictability with both good and bad results from plugs in the same knee.

In an osteochondral defect the ischaemic bone may have been lost from the defect, or it may be incorporated but painful, tender and inflamed as interpreted by bone scan. A 20mm drill will remove this area and provide healthy margins of bone and cartilage. Autologous bone from the medial or lateral femoral condyle can be taken as a tight-fitting plug, inserted into the drilled defect and the surface trimmed to an anatomical level. Autologous chondrocyte implantation using a chondrogide membrane allows reconstruction of overlying cartilage. Alternatively loose graft can be inserted and held in the 'sandwich technique' with a membrane over which ACI is performed.

Fresh osteochondral grafts

Fresh allograft has been highly developed in Toronto. Unfortunately these grafts degenerate over time so that in the surviving transplants (74%) at 15 years over 50% have moderate to severe osteoarthritis despite meniscal transplantation (17%) and concomitant realignment osteotomies to protect the graft (68%). Only 25% of patients at 15 years were known to have a graft that had survived and was not arthritic[1]. What remains to be identified is how well patients proceed with joint replacement following failure of the graft.

Future possibilities

When both bone and cartilage are diseased then both need regenerated. Undertaking this in the loaded situation is difficult. One solution would be to engineer a new joint of cartilage and bone in a bio-reactor in the laboratory. Could a better option be to use the patient as his/her own bioreactor?

This technique is called endo-cultivation and the joint formed an endo-joint. European funding and help from partners across Europe are enabling this project to proceed (www.myjoint.org). A survey of people from across Europe found that over 80% consider this an ethically acceptable use of stem cells.

If endocultivation succeeds it is an option for providing an autologous organ of both bone and cartilage developed to a stage where there is sufficient strength of the engineered tissue to allow early weight-bearing once transplanted into the knee or other joint. In severe situations fresh allograft remains the current best biological option for replacing both diseased bone and cartilage.

References

1. Aubin PP; Cheah HK; Davis AM; Gross AE, Long-term followup of fresh femoral osteochondral allografts for posttraumatic knee defects. Clin Orthop, 2001 Oct, 391 Suppl: S318-27.
2. Akizuki S; Yukihiro Y; Takizawa T, Does arthroscopic abrasion arthroplasty promote cartilage regeneration in osteoarthritic knees with eburnation? A prospective study of high tibial osteotomy with abrasion arthroplasty versus high tibial osteotomy alone. Arthroscopy, 1997, 13 (1): 9-17.
3. Bailey AJ; Mansell JP; Sims TJ; Banse X, Biochemical and mechanical properties of subchondral

bone in osteoarthritis, Biorheology, 2004, 41(3-4): 349-58.

4. Bajada S; Marshall M; Wright K; Richardson J; Johnson W, Decreased osteogenesis, increased cell senescence and elevated Dickkopf-1 secretion in human fracture non union stromal cells, Bone, 2009, 45 (4): 726-735.

5. Bhosale AM; Myint P; Roberts S; Menage J; Harrison P; Ashton B; Smith T; McCall I; Richardson JB, Combined autologous chondrocyte implantation and allogenic meniscus transplantation: A biological knee replacement. The Knee, 2007, 14(5): 361–368.

6. Abhijit Bhosale; Jan Herman Kuiper; W. Eustace B. Johnson; Paul Harrison; James B. Richardson, Midterm to Long-Term Longitudinal Outcome of Autologous Chondrocyte Implantation in the Knee Joint. A Multilevel Analysis, Am J Sports Med, November 2009, 37:131S-138S

7. Carrino JA; Blum J; Parellada JA; Schweitzer ME; Morrison WB, MRI of bone oedema-like signl in he pathogenesis of subchondral cysts, Osteoarthritis and cartilage, October 2006, 14(10): 1081-5.

8. Hulth A, Does osteoarthrosis depend on growth of the mineralized layer of cartilage? Clin Orthop Relat Res, 1993 Feb;(287):19-24.

9. Finsen V, Osteopenia after osteotomy of the tibia, Calcified tissue international, 1987, 42: 1–4.

10. Kelberine F; Frank A, Arthroscopic treatment of osteochondral lesions of the talar dome: a retrospective study of 48 cases. Arthroscopy, 1999, 15(1): 77–84.

11. Kahn M; Kuiper JH; Robinson E; Macdonald L; Bhosale A Richardson JB, Birmingham hip arthroplasty: five to eight years of prospective multicentre follow-up results. J Arthroplasty 2008

12. Luyten FP; Tylzanowski P; Lories RJ, Wnt signaling and osteoarthritis, Bone, April 2009, 44(4): 522-7.

13. Patil S; Butcher W; D'Lima DD; Steklov N; Bugbee WD; Hoenecke HR, Effect of osteochondral graft insertion forces on chondrocyte viability. American Journal of Sports Medicine, 2008 36(9): 1726–32.

14. Pugh JW; Radin EL; Rose RM, Quantitative Studies of Human Subchondral Cancellous Bone J Bone Joint Surg Am, 1974, 56:313-321.

15. Raynauld JP; Martel-Pelletier J; Berthiaume MJ; Abram F; Choquette D; Haraoui B; Beary JF, Cline GA; Meyer JM; Pelletier JP, Correlation between bone lesion changes and cartilage volume loss in patients with osteoarthritis of the knee as assessed by quantitative magnetic resonance imaging over a 24 month period. Annals of Rheumatic Diseases, May 2008, 67(5): 683-8.

16. Sabokbar A; Crawford R; Murray DW; Athanasou NA, Macrophage-osteoclast differentiation and bone resorption in osteoarthrotic subchondral acetabular cysts, Acta Orthopaedica Scandinavica, June 2000, 71(3): 255-61.

17. Sharpe JR; Ahmed SU; Fleetcroft JP; Martin R, The treatment of osteochondral lesions using a combination of autologous chondrocyte implantation and autograft: three-year follow-up, J Bone Joint Surg Br, 2005 May, 87(5):730-5.

18. Schultz W; Gobel D, Articular cartilage regeneration of the knee joint after proximal tibial valgus osteotomy: a prospective study of different intra- and extra-articular operative techniques, Knee Surg Sports Traumatol Arthrosc, 1999, 7:29.

19. Smith GD; Laing PW; Makwana N; Roberts S; Richardson JB, Autologous chondrocyte implantation in the ankle: clinical results up to 10 years. Poster abstracted P188, ICRS 2009.

20. Stukenborg-Colsman C; Wirth CJ; Lazovic D; Wefer A, High tibial osteotomy versus unicompartmental joint replacement in unicompartmental knee joint osteoarthritis: 7-10-year follow-up prospective randomised study, Knee, 2001 Oct, 8(3): 187-94.

21. Spahn G, Complications in high tibial osteotomy, Archives of Orthopaedic and Trauma Surgery, 2004, 124: 649–653.

22. Van der Vis; Harm M; Aspenberg P; Marti RK; Tigchelaar W; Van Noorden C, Fluid pressure causes resorption in a rabbit model of prosthetic loosening. Clin Orth and Rel Res, 1998, 350: 201–208.

23. Wade RH; New AMR; Tselentakis G; Kuiper JH; Roberts A; Richardson JB, Malunion in the Lower Limb - A Nomogram to Predict the Effects of Osteotomy. Journal of Bone and Joint Surgery, March 1999, 81B(2): 312-316.

24. Wang H; Kandel RA, Chondrocytes attach to hyaline or calcified cartilage and bone, Osteoarthritis and Cartilage, Jan 2004, 12(1): 56-64.

"Some patients, though conscious that their condition is perilous, recover their health simply through their contentment with the goodness of the physician"

(Hippocrates 460-400 B.C.)

CHAPTER 7.

BIOMATERIALS AND CARTILAGE REPAIR

Elizaveta Kon, Marco Delcogliano, Alessandro Di Martino, Giuseppe Filardo, Giuliana Niceforo, Viviana Zarbà, Stefano Zaffagnini, Maurilio Marcacci

---

Take Home Message

A good biomaterial for cartilage repair should ideally be:
1. *An off-the-shelf graft in a one-step surgical procedure.*
2. *From a surgical standpoint, it should be inserted under minimally invasive conditions.*
3. *Should be a graded biomimetic osteochondral scaffold, promoting by itself bone and cartilage tissue restoration by inducing selective bone marrow stem cell differentiation in osteogenic and chondrogenic lineages.*

Introduction

The use of biomaterials for cartilage repair has strongly increased in the last decade, due to promising results obtained with the development of new therapeutic options for the treatment of articular cartilage lesions. Actually in clinical practice there are two main concepts for biomaterials application for cartilage repair: cartilage regeneration promoted by cultured autologous chondrocytes, supported by the 3D scaffold (so-called second generation autologous chondrocyte transplantation) or implant of various biomaterials for "in situ" cartilage repair which exploits bone marrow stem cess differentiation induced by the scaffold properties.

The use of classic ACI (first generation) has been associated with several limitations related to the complexity and the morbidity of the surgical procedure. To address these problems so-called second generation ACI techniques have been developed. The second generation ACI used a tissue-engineering technology to create a cartilage-like tissue in a three-dimensional culture system with the attempt to address all the concerns related to the cell culture and the surgical technique. Essentially, the concept is based on the use of biodegradable polymers as temporary scaffolds for the in vitro growth of living cells and their subsequent transplantation onto the defect site. Essential properties of these scaffolds include biocompatibility and biodegradability through safe biochemical pathways at suitable time intervals. It is known that chondrocytes in two-dimensional cell cultures alter their phenotype and dedifferentiate to fibroblast cells that no longer posses the capacity to produce collagen type II and proteglycans. The use of three-dimensional scaffolds has been shown to favor the maintenance of a chondrocyte differentiated phenotype[1,2]. The clinical application of this second generation tissue engineered approach is well documented for different types of scaffold with an evaluation of the clinical outcome at short and medium-term follow up[3,4,5,6].

Biomaterials associated with Chondrocyte Transplantation: 2nd generation ACI Autologous chondrocyte transplantation on a three-dimensional matrix was introduced in clinical practice in Europe from 1998-1999, so it is very difficult to obtain long-term clinical findings. Matrixes mainly used in clinical practice in Europe are collagen or hyaluronic acid based.

In 1998 Behrens and Steinwachs et al performed the first auotologous chondrocytes transplantation using a porcine collagen type I/III membrane (Chondro-Gide, Geistlich Biomaterilas, Switzerland) with MACI technique as a scaffold to enable treatment of larger defects that can be hard to treat with standard microfracturing alone. Autologous chondrocytes were directly inoculated onto type I/III collagen membrane and delivered as a cell scaffold construct for implantation (MACT, MACI®, Verigen Transplantation Service, Copenhagen, Denmark). The surgical procedure as every procedures named as 2 generation ACI comprehends two surgery steps: the harvesting of articular cartilage from a non weight bearing area and, in a second operative procedure, the arthrotomic implant of the MACI® into the defect. In the while between the procedures the cells are cultured subsequently for 4 weeks before being seeded on the rough side of the porcine collagen type I/III matrix, the loaded matrix is then cultured with autologous serum for the remaining 3 days. Since the introduction of the MACI® technique in 1998, more than 3000 patients have been treated across Europe and Australia[7,8]. Hyalograft C® was introduced into clinical practice in a number of European countries in 1999 for the treatment of full-thickness cartilage defects. This scaffold is entirely based on the benzylic ester of hyaluronic acid (HYAFF® 11, Fidia Advanced Biopolymers Laboratories, Padova, Italy) and consists of a network of 20-μm-thick fibers with interstices of variable sizes. The cells harvested from the patient are expanded and then seeded onto the scaffold to create the tissue-engineered product Hyalograft C®. Seeded on the scaffold the cells are able to re-differentiate and retain a chondrocytic phenotype even after a long period of in vitro expansion in monolayer culture[4].

The features of this device have also permitted the development of an arthroscopic surgical technique for implantation of autologous chondrocytes on a hyaluronic acid support with the aim of reducing patient morbidity, surgical time and recovery and complications related to open surgery[9].

The results using Hyalograft C® are comparable with the ones of the original ACI technique[10].

Lately many interesting scaffold have been proposed in preclinical studies; only a few have been introduced in the clinical practice, though.

Nehrer at al.[11] explored a novel matrix-based implant cartilage repair composed of both fibrin and hyaluronan in a defined ratio that takes advantage of the biological and mechanical properties of these two elements. The matrix was seeded with autologous chondrocytes expanded in the presence of a proprietary growth factor variant designed to preserve their chondrogenic potential. They prospectively followed eight patients with symptomatic-chronic cartilage defects treated with this 2 steps procedure. The clinical outcome of a 1-year follow-up demonstrated increase of clinical scores. The MRI follow-up showed good filling of the defect with tissue having the imaging appearance of cartilage in all patients.

Kreuz at al.[12] evaluated the Clinical outcome after four-year clinical follow-up of 19 patients treated with Bioseed C®, a cell-based cartilage graft based on autologous chondrocytes embedded in fibrin and a stable resorbable polymer scaffold. Significant improvement ($p<0.05$) of the Lysholm and the ICRS score was observed as early as 6 months after implantation of BioSeed (R)-C and remained stable during follow-up.

Selmi TA et al.[13] investigated the clinical, radiological, arthroscopic and histological outcome at a minimum follow-up of two years after the implantation of autologous chondrocytes embedded in a three-dimensional alginate-agarose hydrogel Cartipatch® (TBF Banque de tissues, France) for the treatment of chondral and osteochondral defects. Clinically, all the 17 patients treated improved significantly. Patients with lesions larger than 3 cm^2 improved significantly more than those with smaller lesions.

Matrix-associated chondrocyte implantation has been used with promising results in Europe and Australia but is not routinely available in the United States where there is not FDA approval for matrix-assisted chondrocyte transplantation in human application, yet.

Therefore a different and new approach has been developed to avoid the problems related to the ex vivo chondrocyte culture and expansion in a scaffold. In this technique, healthy cartilage tissue is harvested from an unaffected area of the injured joint and mechanically fragmented. The cartilage fragments are then embedded into a 3-Dpolymeric resorbable scaffold,which is then implanted into the auricular cartilage defect (CartilageAutograft ImplantationSystem CAIS, J&J Regeneration Technologies, Raynham, MA). Experimental studies have demonstrated that out growth and migration of chondrocytes from the implanted cartilage fragments result in chondrocyte redistribution within the scaffold and produce hyaline-like repair tissue at 6 months[14]. Clinical studies have shown the safety of this procedure and randomized, multi-center studies are currently under way to evaluate the clinical efficiency of this approach[15]. This novel approach assails one of the more discussed disadvantage related to the second-generation ACI procedures. In fact, even though these procedures reduce morbidity and avoid the use of a periosteal flap with marked advantages from a biological and surgical point of view obtaining results comparable and even better of the Classic ACI technique[11], the 2nd Generation ACI techniques remain related to all the problems of cells culture: cost-effectiveness and two steps surgery.

"On shelf" Biomaterials

Considering that from a surgical and commercial standpoint, an ideal graft for chondral or osteochondral defect repair would be an off-the-shelf product; thus, some new biomaterials were recently proposed to induce "in situ" cartilage regeneration after direct transplantation onto the defect site. The possibility to create a cell-free implant to be sufficiently "intelligent" to bring into the joint the appropriate cues to induce orderly and durable tissue regeneration is still under investigation in numerous animal studies[16-22], but only few of these have been introduced into the clinical practice[23,24].

Scaffolds composed of synthetic or natural materials in a variety of physical forms (fibers, meshes, gels) have been used for cartilage regeneration. Solid scaffolds provide a substrate upon which cells may adhere, while gel scaffolds function to physically entrap the cells. Commonly used synthetic materials are the polylactides, like polylactic (PLA) and polyglicolic (PGA) acids. The mechanical properties and the degradation of synthetic biomaterials are more easily modified that for the natural polymers, but their degradation products may cause damage to native tissue or implanted cells. However new chemistry of these materials has improved their biocharacteristic and biocompatibility. Natural materials used to produce scaffolds include agarose, alginate, hyaluronic acid, gelatin, fibrin glue, collagen derivatives and acellular collagen matrix. They have impeccable biocompatibility, can be processed in a reliable and reproducible way and may enhance cell performance. The materials mostly used actually in clinical practice are protein-based (collagen or gelatine), but the use of polysaccharides is in rapid growth. There are several studies pointing to the critical role of saccharide molecules in cell signalling schemes and their importance in cartilage regeneration[25,26]. One of the more important properties of polysaccharides in general is their ability to form hydrogels. Hydrogel formation can occur by a number of mechanisms and is strongly influenced by the types of monosaccharide involved: for example thermal gellation is tipical for agarose and pH-dependent gellation for chitosan. Chitosan (partially de-acetylated derivative of chitin, found in arthropod exoskeletons) seems to have an important potential in stimulating chondrogenesis[26] and there are some chitosan-based gels and scaffolds under clinical investigation for "in situ" cartilage regeneration after direct transplantation onto the defect site.

The treatment of large osteochondral articular defects represents a relevant problem in orthopaedic practice.

Actually, no tissue engineered constructs for osteochondral transplantation are available for clinical use. The treatment of osteochondral lesions is biologically challenging since two different tissues are involved (bone and articular cartilage) with a distinctly different intrinsic healing capacity. There are some composite materials in pre-clinical and clinical experimentation for tissue engineered and "in situ" regeneration approach for cartilage repair.

Niederauer GG et al.[16] prepared a multiphase implant prototypes using poly(D,L) lactide-co-glycolide as the base material. PGA fibers (FR), 45S5 Bioglass (BG) and medical grade calcium sulfate (MGCS) were used as additives to vary stiffness and chemical properties. Osteochondral defects were treated in the medial femoral condyle (high-weight bearing) and the distal medial portion of the patellar groove (low-weight bearing) of Spanish goats. Half of the implants were loaded with autologous chondrocytes. Qualitative evaluations showed that all groups had a high percentage of hyaline cartilage and good bony restoration, with new tissue integrating well with the native cartilage; no difference in healing for implant types or addition/omission of cells was found.

Buma et al.[17] implanted cross-linked type I and type II collagen matrices, with and without attached chondroitin sulfate, into full-thickness defects in the femoral trochlea of adolescent rabbits. The tissue response was evaluated 4 and 12 weeks after implantation by general histology and two semi-quantitative histological grading systems. Four weeks after implantation, type I collagenous matrices were completely filled withcartilage-like tissue. By contrast, type II collagenous matrices revealed predominantly cartilaginous tissue only at the superficial zone and at the interface of the matrix with the subchondral bone, leaving large areas of the matrix devoid of tissue. Attachment of chondroitin sulfate appeared to promote cellular ingrowth and cartilaginous tissue formation in both types of collagen matrices.

Hoeman et al[18] filled with chitosan-glycerol phosphate/autologous blood a cartilage defect treated with microfracture in fourteen sheep. At six months, defects that had been treated with chitosan-glycerol phosphate/blood were filled with significantly more hyaline repair tissue ($p < 0.05$) compared with control defects.

Jiang et al.[19] developed a biphasic cylindrical porous plug of DL-poly-lactide-co-glycolide, with its lower body impregnated with B-tricalciumphosphate as the osseous phase. They tested the clinical applicability of such composite construct implanting it, cell-free and seeded with autologous condrocytes, in the femoral condyles of Lee-Sung mini-pigs. Six months after surgery they found good scaffold integration with cancellous bone formed in the implant periphery. In the chondral phase, hyaline cartilage regeneration was found in cell-seeded group whereas only fibrous tissue formed in the control group.

Nagura et al.[20] developed a PLG bio-absorbable porous scaffold (Pelham, Alabama) and tested it on full-thickness osteochondral defect in rabbit. The absorption of scaffold with regeneration of osteochondral defect was noted. They supposed that a balance between the porosity and pore size play a important role for both restoration and remodeling of cartilage and bone and degradation of PLG scaffold.

Schlichting et al.[21] reported the osteochondral defect healing using a polyactide-co-glycolide copolymer with calcium sulfate scaffold (PolyGraft, OsteoBiologies Inc, San Antonio, Texas) in two group of sheep. One group was treated with a stiff scaffold and the group with a modified softer one. A better healing of osteochondral defect with stiff scaffold was detected.

Schagemann et al.[22] carried out the study on osteochondral repair treated with implantation of cell-laden and cell-free alginate-gelatin biopolymer hydrogel in sheep. Four femoral defects per animal were filled with hydrogel plus autologous chondrocytes or periosteal cells or gel only or were left untreated. Defects after hydrogel plus autologous chondrocytes were restored with smooth, hyaline-like neo-cartilage and trabecular subchondral bone. Gel only treatment revealed slightly inferior regenerate morphology.

However, in spite of all the pre-clinical studies reported, only one scaffold used for osteochondral regeneration is commercialized for clinical application. This is a bilayer porous PLGA-calcium-solfate biopolymer (TruFit). Although pre-clinical experimentation is promising[15] there are still no systematic controlled studies, only isolated reports have shown favourable results after implantation of these osteochondral graft substitutes[15, 23]. However, MRI information at 12 months still demonstrated heterogeneous repair cartilage tissue and information on long term durability is not available[23].

Another interesting cell-free approach is represented by a technique that combines the microfracturing with the application of a porcine collagen type-III/I bi-layer matrix to stabilise the blood clot. AMIC® as 1-step procedure enables the reasonable treatment of larger (>2 cm²) cartilage defects. Steinwachs reports promising clinical results of the first 32 patients associated with a good defect filling in MRI[24].

Rizzoli experience

We utilized an osteochondral nanostructured biomimetic scaffold (Fin-Ceramica S.p.A., Faenza - Italy) with a porous 3-D tri-layer composite structure, mimicking the whole osteochondral anatomy. The cartilaginous layer, consisting of Type I collagen, has a smooth surface to favour the joint flow. The intermediate layer (tide-mark-like) consists of a combination of Type I collagen (60%) and HA (40%), whereas the lower layer consists of a mineralized blend of Type I collagen (30%) and HA (70%) reproducing the sub-chondral bone layer.

In vitro and animal studies showed good results in terms of both cartilage and bone tissue formation. We observed same macroscopic, histological and radiographic results when implanting scaffold loaded with autologous chondrocytes or scaffold alone. The scaffold was able to induce an in situ regeneration through stem cells coming from the surrounding bone marrow[27,28,29]. Thus, we applied this innovative scaffold as a cell-free approach into clinical practice.

We have performed a clinical pilot study on 30 patients where the newly developed scaffold was used for the treatment of chondral and osteochondral lesions of the knee joint in order to evaluate the safety and the reproducibility of the surgical procedure and in order to test the intrinsic potential of the device. The clinical outcome of all patients was analyzed prospectively, at 6 months and 1 year, and with a high resolution MRI. 29 of 30 patients (mean age of 29.3 years) were prospectively evaluated at 6 and 12 months follow-up (one patient lost at follow-up). In 29 patients 35 lesions were treated, average size of the defects was 2.8 cm² (range: 1.5– 5.9 cm²).

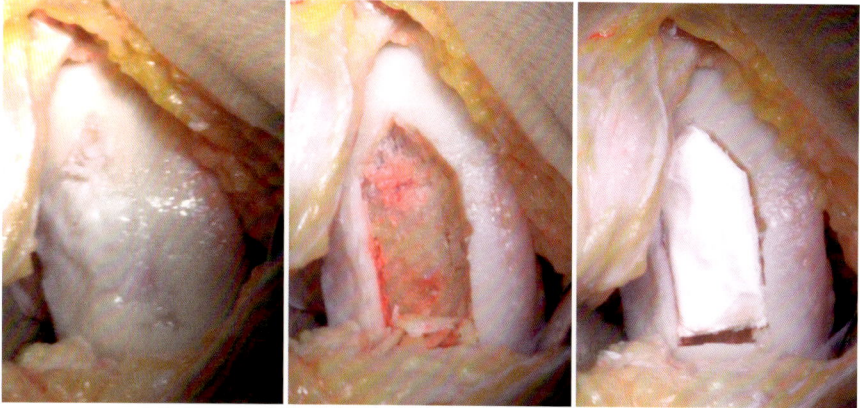

Figure 1: Novel osteochondral scaffold: intraoperative view

Statistical analysis demonstrated a significant improvement (Non Parametric paired Wilcoxon test, p<0.0005) from pre-operative to 12 months follow-up. IKDC objective score showed preoperatively 46.1% of normal or nearly normal knees and 79.3% of normal or nearly normal knees at 12 months. Statistical analysis showed a significant improvement in the IKDC subjective score from pre-operative (37.5±14.6) to 12 months follow-up (82.4±11.9) (Non Parametric paired Wilcoxon test, p<0.0005).

MRI evaluation showed: complete filling of cartilage defect was noted in 86.2% of the patients and the congruency of the articular surface was seen in same patients. Subchondral bone changes (edema or sclerosis) were noted in 53.3% of patients.

This scaffold, composed of Type-I collagen and nanostructured hydroxyapatite, was designed for the treatment of cartilaginous and osteocartilaginous defects and have demonstrated to stimulate in situ bone and cartilage regeneration. Obviously, this short follow-up does not allow us to draw conclusions about the clinical effectiveness and histological quality of cartilage repair tissue in the long-term follow-up of this procedure, but clinical and MRI analysis allowed us to study and better understand the potential of this novel developed scaffold. The ability of the scaffold to induce orderly osteochondral tissue repair without necessarily including autologous cells makes it attractive (i) from a practical standpoint, since it could be used as an off-the-shelf graft in a one-step surgical procedure, (ii) from a surgical standpoint, since due to its flexibility it could inserted under minimally invasive conditions. Previous animal study highlighted the good potential of the graded biomimetic osteochondral scaffold in promoting by itself bone and cartilage tissue restoration, probably by inducing selective bone marrow stem cell differentiation in osteogenic and chondrogenic lineages[29]. Further systematic evaluation is necessary to determine the clinical and morphological outcome, especially compared to other treatment options such as bone-marrow stimulation techniques, mosaicplasty, and autologous chondrocyte transplantation.

Acknowledgement

Angela Montaperto, Laura Bragonzoni, Elettra Pignotti, Keith Smith, Istituto Orto-
pedico Rizzoli, Bologna, Italy.
This study was realized with financial contribution of European Project
"TemPlant".

References

1. Grigolo B; Lisignoli G; Piacentini A; et al., Evidence for redifferentiation of human chondrocytes grown on a hyaluronan-based biomaterial (HYAff 11): molecular, immunohistochemical and ultrastructural analysis, Biomaterials, 2002 Feb, 23(4):1187-95
2. Freed LE; Marquis JC ; Nohria A ; et al., Neocartilage formation in vitro and in vivo using cells cultured on synthetic biodegradable polymers, J Biomed Mater Res, 1993 Jan, 27(1):11-23
3. Kon E; Delcogliano M; Filardo G; Montaperto C; Marcacci M, Second generation issue in cartilage repair, Sports Med Arthrosc, 2008 Dec,16(4):221-9
4. Behrens P; Bitter T; Kurz B; et al., Matrix-associated autologous chondrocyte transplantation/implantation (MATC/MACI)-5-year follow –up, The knee, 2006,13:194-202
5. Nehrer S; Domayer S; Dorotka R; et al., Three-year clinical outcome after chondrocyte transplantation using a hyaluronan matrix for cartilage repair, European Journal of Radiology, 2006, 57:3-8
6. Kon E; Gobbi A; Filardo G; Delcogliano M; Zaffagnini S; Marcacci M; Arthroscopic second-generation autologous chondrocyte implantation compared with microfracture for chondral lesions of the knee: prospective nonrandomized study at 5 years, Am J Sports Med, 2009 Jan, 37(1):33-41
7. Behrens P; Bitter T; Kurz B; et al. Matrix-associated autologous chondrocyte transplantation/implantation (MATC/MACI)-5-year follow –up, The knee, 2006, 13:194-202
8. Zheng MH; Willers C; Wood D, Matrix-induced autologous chondrocytes implantation (MACI®): biological and clinical evaluation. Basic science, clinical repair and reconstruction of articular cartilage defects: Current status and prospects. Chapter 54, 2006, 517-528
9. Marcacci M; Zaffagnini S; Kon E; et al., Arthroscopic autologous chondrocyte transplantation: technical note, Knee Surg Sports Traumatol Arthrosc, 2002 May, 10(3):154-9
10. Ferruzzi A; Buda R; Faldini C; Vannini F; Di Caprio F; Luciani D; Giannini S, Autologous chondrocyte implantation in the knee joint: open compared with arthroscopic technique. Comparison at a minimum follow-up of five years, J Bone Joint Surg Am, 2008 Nov, 90 Suppl 4:90-101
11. Nehrer S; Chiari C; Domayer S; Barkay H; Yayon A, Results of chondrocyte implantation with a fibrin-hyaluronan matrix: a preliminary study, Clin Orthop Relat Res, 2008 Aug, 466(8):1849-55
12. Kreuz PC; Muller S; Ossendorf C; Kaps C; Erggelet C, Treatment of focal degenerative cartilage defects with polymer-based autologous chondrocyte grafts: four year clinical results, Arthritis Res Ther, 2009 Mar 5,11(2):R33
13. Selmi TA; Verdonk P; Chambat P; Dubrana F; Potel JF; Barnouin L; Neyret P, Autologous chondrocyte implantation in a novel alginate-agarose hydrogel: outcome at two years, J Bone Joint Surg Br, 2008 May, 90(5):597-604
14. Lu Y; Dhanaraj S; Wang Z; et al, Minced cartilage without cell colcture serves as an effective cell source for cartilage repair, J Orthop Research, 2006, 24: 1261-70
15. Mithoefer K; McAdams TR; Scopp JM; Mandelbaum BR, Emerging options for treatment of articular cartilage injury in the athlete, Clin Sports Med, 2009 Jan, 28(1):25-40
16. Niederauer GG; Slivka MA; Leatherbury NC; Korvick DL; Harroff HH; Ehler WC; et al., Evaluation of multiphase implants for repair of focal osteochondral defects in goats, Biomaterials, 2000, 21: 2561-74
17. Buma P; Pieper JS; van Tienen T; van Susante JLC; van der Kraan PM; Veerkamp JH; et al., Cross-linked type I and type II collagenous matrices for the repair of full-thickness articular cartilage defects: a study in rabbits, Biomaterials, 2003, 24: 3255-63
18. Hoemann CD; Hurtig M; Rossomacha E; Sun J; Chevrier A; Shive MS; et al., Chitosan-glycerol phosphate/blood implants improve hyaline cartilage repair in ovine microfracture defects, J Bone Joint Surg Am, 2005, 87: 2671-86
19. Jiang CC; Chiang H; Liao CJ; et al., Repair of porcine articular cartilage defect with a biphasic

osteochondral composite, J Orthop Res, 2007 Oct, 25(10):1277-90

20. Nagura I; Fujioka H; Kokubu T; Makino T; Sumi Y; Kurosaka M, Repair of osteochondral defects with a new porous synthetic polymer scaffold, J Bone Joint Surg Br, 2007 Feb, 89(2):258-64

21. Schlichting K; Schell H; Kleemann RU; Schill A; Weiler A; Duda GN; Epari DR, Influence of scaffold stiffness on subchondral bone and subsequent cartilage regeneration in an ovine model of osteochondral defect healing, Am J Sports Med, 2008 Dec, 36(12):2379-91

22. Schagemann JC; Erggelet C; Chung HW; Lahm A; Kurz H; Mrosek EH, Cell-Laden and Cell-Free Biopolymer Hydrogel for the Treatment of Osteochondral Defects in a Sheep Model, Tissue Eng Part A, 2008 Sep 10

23. Williams RJ; Gamradt SC, Articular cartilage repair using a resorbable matrix scaffold, AAOS Instr Course lect, 2008, 57:563-71

24. Steinwachs MR; Guggi T; Kreuz PC, Marrow stimulation techniques, Injury, 2008 Apr, 39 Suppl 1:S26-31

25. Suh JK; Matthew HW, Application of chitosan-based polysaccharide biomaterials in cartilage tissue engineering: a review, Biomaterials, 2000 Dec, 21(24):2589-98

26. Hoemann CD; Sun J; McKee MD; Chevrier A; Rossomacha E; Rivard GE; Hurtig M; Buschmann MD, Chitosan-glycerol phosphate/blood implants elicit hyaline cartilage repair integrated with porous subchondral bone in microdrilled rabbit defects, Osteoarthritis Cartilage, 2007 Jan,15(1):78-89

27. Tampieri A; Celotti G; Landi E; Sandri M; Roveri N; Falini G, Biologically inspired synthesis of bone-like composite: self-assembled collagen fibers/hydroxyapatite nanocrystals, J Biomed Mater Res A, 2003, 67: 618-25

28. Tampieri A; Sandri M; Landi E; Pressato D; Francioli S; Quarto R; Martin I, Design of graded Biomimetic osteochondral composite scaffold, Biomaterials, 2008 Sep, 29(26):3539-46

29. Kon E; Delcogliano M; Filardo G; Fini M; Giavaresi G; Franciol Si; Martin I; Pressato D; Arcangeli E; Quarto R; Sandri M; and Marcacci M, Orderly osteochondral regeneration in a sheep model using a novel nano-composite multi biomaterial, J Orthop Res, 2010 Jan, 28(1):116-24

"We make all the calculations, the patients takes the risks"

(Peter Marcello, 2002)

Chapter 8.

Cartilage Repair Treatment Flow Charts

Bert R. Mandelbaum, Jason Boyer, Marco Delcogliano

Take Home Message

- *Marrow stimulation techniques, substitution replacement options and biologic replacement options each have a role in the treatment algorithm of articular cartilage defects.*
- *When using a treatment algorithm one must take into account not only the characterization of the specific cartilage lesion but also the myriad of local and regional factors as well as the co-morbidities attached to each patient.*
- *Still no single treatment option can re-establish the hyaline cartilage seen in normal articular cartilage.*

Introduction

The clinical consequences of articular cartilage defects of the knee are pain, swelling, mechanical symptoms, athletic and functional disability and osteoarthritis. Full thickness articular cartilage defects have a poor capacity to heal, due to the cartilage's isolation from systemic regulation and its lack of vessels and nerve supply. The challenge to restore the articular cartilage surface is a multidimensional task faced by both basic scientists in the laboratory and orthopedic surgeons in the operating room. A growing number of patients are presenting for consultation in order to maintain their active lifestyles and hobbies. These patients wish to continue activities that have, in the past, been achievable only for younger and healthier knees. In the last 30 years, different techniques to address articular cartilage injuries and defects have emerged as valid therapeutic options. While options to treat these lesions have expanded, the difficulty facing practitioners is choosing which technique to best address the defects of each individual patient.

While the regeneration of true hyaline cartilage is not yet reality, a variety of methods have the potential to stimulate the formation of a new articular surface, including microfracture of subchondral bone, use of auto and/or allografts, cell transplantation, targeted growth factors and artificial matrices. Reports of the clinical results of these procedures have documented clinical improvement for most of the patients[1,2,3,4]. However, despite the availability of all of these techniques and the advances in imaging that have led to an increased understanding of the frequency and types of chondral lesions, patient evaluation and treatment selection still remain challenging. In evaluating a patient for cartilage repair, one must characterize not only the cartilage lesion itself, but the various clinical factors and co-morbidities embodied by each individual.

Several co-morbidities such as ligamentous instability, deficient menisci or malalignment of the mechanical limb axis or extensor mechanism often coexist with the articular surface pathology. Moreover age-related, non –progressive, superficial fibrillation of cartilage and focal lesions of the articular surface must be distinguished from degeneration of cartilage occurring as a part of syndrome of osteoarthritis[5]. As a consequence, the clinician must define, characterize and classify local, regional and systemic, medical and family history factors that may influence the progression, degeneration or regeneration of the defect. Careful patient evaluation is essential in selecting the proper treatment plan: lesions with different etiology and size require different treatments and the co-morbidities may need to be treated in conjunction with symptomatic chondral injuries to provide a mutually beneficial effect. Thus, the evaluation and characterization of the patient as a whole is key to optimizing the results of surgery.

The purpose of this chapter is to provide the guidelines to select the proper treatment algorithm.

Clinical Management

The initial step in the workup is the history. This should include mechanism of injury, time course and quality of symptoms and review of previous treatment and the effects of those treatments. Peterson et al found that the average patient presenting for cartilage restoration had 2.1 previous treatments, usually with a different physician[6]. In this setting, access to operative reports, pervious imaging and even direct communication with previously treating surgeons can provide information.

During the physical examination, the surgeon should be careful not to assume that the articular cartilage lesion is responsible for all symptoms, but should attempt to delineate concomitant pathologies that may be contributing symptoms. It is important to recognize that not all chondral lesions cause symptoms. Conversely, not all symptoms are related to the chondral or osteochondral defect. Often concomitant pathology exists and can play a role in the symptoms that the patient maybe experiencing. In addition to the sites of point tenderness, effusion, crepitus and catching, the examination should carefully assess alignment, range of motion and patellofemoral tracking. Evaluation for ligamentous integrity is also valuable in considering concomitant pathologies of the knee. Other mechanical issues of obesity and gait patterns may exclude a patient from certain treatments because of potential inability to comply with often extensive rehabilitation protocols.

Required radiographs include standing anteroposterior, lateral, patellar skyline, a 45 degree flexion posterior anterior weight-bearing view and a full length alignment film. No cartilage restoration procedure should be performed in the setting of malalignment; therefore, if the mechanical axis bisects the affected compartment, a corrective osteotomy should be strongly considered as a concomitant or staged procedure[7,8].

Access to MRI is important in developing and executing an effective clinical approach to cartilage repair surgery. With a high-resolution fast spin echo sequencing technique in the sagital, coronal, and axial planes, articular cartilage surfaces can be well imaged and measured. This allows accurate characterization of not only the lesions in question, but the state of all opposing cartilage surfaces and menisci. Quantitative MRI techniques, such as T2 mapping, T1 rho, and delayed gadolinium-enhanced MRI of cartilage (dGEMRIC), provide noninvasive information about cartilage and repair tissue biochemistry. Diffusion-weighted imaging (DWI) and diffusion tensor imaging (DTI) demonstrate information regarding the regional anisotropic variation of cartilage ultrastructure9.These advantages provide preoperative information and may allow for a postoperative assessment of actual glycosaminoglycan content of repaired or replaced tissue[10]. If the lesion involves the subchondral bone then computer tomography scanning may also be necessary to assess defect geometry and depth, especially in the presence of osteochondral defects that may require bone grafting in addition to an articular cartilage restorative procedure.

An examination under anesthesia is required to better assess the knee instability. This is performed routinely prior to every knee arthroscopy. The first operation after the diagnosis of an articular cartilage defect is often not the definitive procedure. At times, arthroscopy is performed initially as a diagnostic tool to assess the lesion, in terms of its location, geography, surface area and depth. The surrounding articular surfaces in the uninvolved compartments, the state of the menisci and the presence or absence of additional pathology need also to be defined. If one is considering definitive treatment with ACI, a biopsy should be performed at this time. Similarly, if a significant subchondral defect exists; primary bone grafting can be performed at the index operation.

Local and regional factors

To ensure uniform standards of evaluating articular cartilage repair, a universally accepted classification system is necessary. Many different grading systems for cartilage defects are cited in the literature including those of Outerbridge[11], Insall[12], Bauer and Jackson[13], and Noyes and Stobler[14]. To avoid confusion, the International Cartilage Repair Society has developed a grading system to be used as a universal language when surgeons are communicating about cartilage lesions. The ICRS characterizes changes as normal as Grade 0, Grade 1 as softening, Grade II as fibrillation, Grade III as fissuring and Grade IV as reaching the depth of bone (Figure 1).

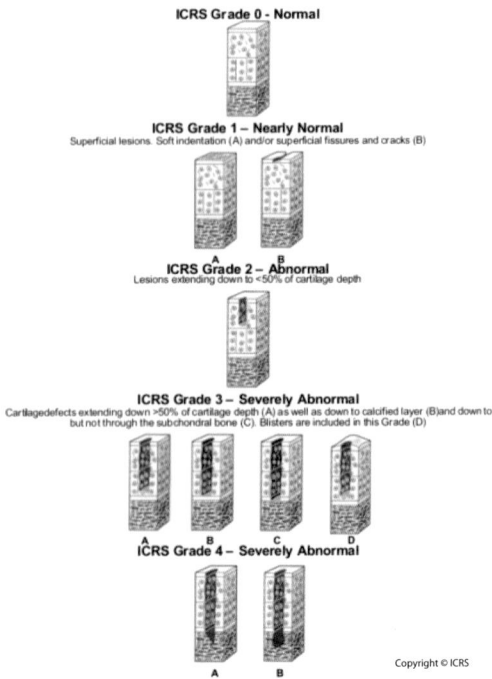

ICRS Grade 0 - Normal

ICRS Grade 1 – Nearly Normal
Superficial lesions. Soft indentation (A) and/or superficial fissures and cracks (B)

ICRS Grade 2 – Abnormal
Lesions extending down to <50% of cartilage depth

ICRS Grade 3 – Severely Abnormal
Cartilage defects extending down >50% of cartilage depth (A) as well as down to calcified layer (B) and down to but not through the subchondral bone (C). Blisters are included in this Grade (D)

ICRS Grade 4 – Severely Abnormal

Copyright © ICRS

Images reproduced with authorization from the International Cartilage Repair Society - ICRS

Figure 1: ICRS criteria for grading of chondral lesions.

This grading system is also included in a comprehensive method of documentation and classification which encompasses a global description of not only the lesion but all of the local factors and co-morbidities previously discussed[15]. The following variables are included in the standards.
• Etiology. Is the defect acute or chronic? This may be a difficult differentiation since there is a blend of acute and chronic and combinations.
• Defect Thickness. What is the thickness or depth of the defect as defined by

the ICRS grade? (Figure 1). Penetration of the tidemark and/or the presence of subchondral cysts can affect the functional articular cartilage unit.

• Lesion size. A probe accurately measures size in centimeters squared during arthroscopy. Defects less than 2 cm^2 have different treatment options than defects greater than 2 cm^2.

• Degree of containment. Is the defect contained or uncontained? Is the surrounding articular cartilage healthy or degenerative? As the degree of containment decreases, consequent loss of joint space is seen on radiographs

• Location. Is the defect in the weight-bearing region of the knee? Is it monopolar or bipolar?

• Ligamentous integrity. Are the cruciate ligaments intact, partially torn or completely torn? Is there residual instability or has the knee been reconstructed?

• Meniscal integrity. Are the menisci intact? If not, has there been a partial, subtotal or complete meniscectomy? Has meniscal repair or transplantation been performed?

• Alignment. Is the alignment normal, varus or valgus? Is there patellofemoral malalignment? Has an osteotomy or realignment procedure been performed?

• Dynamic Alignment.

• Previous management. If a prior cartilage restorative procedure has been performed, was the subchondral plate violated?

• Radiological assessment. Weight bearing AP or flexed PA views, lateral views and patellofemoral views are necessary for the evaluation of joint space narrowing and subchondral cyst formation.

• MRI assessment. New MRI sequences allow for the preoperative and postoperative evaluation of defects and articular cartilage repairs. Bone bruising, osteochondritis dissecans and avascular necrosis can also be evaluated.

• General medical, systemic and family history issues. Is there a rheumatologic history? Are there endocrine related factors? Is there a family history of osteoarthritis or cartilage disorders?

A comprehensive analysis of the local and regional factors related to an articular cartilage lesion is utilized to develop a treatment plan. A flow chart has been created to summarize primary treatment options and secondary treatment options. There are separate charts for femoral and for patellar defects. Primary treatment options should be considered first line treatment choices. Secondary treatment options are considered if primary treatment fails or if other factors prevent the use of a primary treatment option. (Figure 2, Figure 3).

FEMORAL DEFECTS

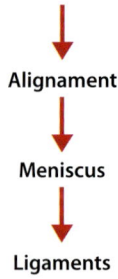

↓

Alignament

↓

Meniscus

↓

Ligaments

1° Treatment Options

Size	Small 0-1cm	Medium 1-2cm	Large >2cm
Microfracture	++	++	+?
O.C.G.	++	++	-
Allograft	--	--	++
A.C.I.	--	--	++
A.C.I 2	--	--	++

2° Treatment Options

Size	Small 0-1cm	Medium 1-2cm	Large >2cm
Microfracture	++	+	-
O.C.G.	++	++	-
Allograft	-	-	++
A.C.I.	-	++	++
A.C.I 2	-	++	++

Legend
-   Treatment not recommended
+   Acceptable treatment
++ Optimal treatment

Figure 2.

TROCHLEAR and/or PATELLAR DEFECTS

↓

Alignament

1° Treatment Options

Size	Small <2cm	Large >2cm
Rehabilitation	++	++
Microfracture	++	++
Lateral Release	+	+

2° Treatment Options

Size	Small 0-1cm	Large >2cm
A.C.I	+	++
A.C.I 2	+	++
Allograft	-	++
Lateral Release	+	+
P.F. Realignment	+	++

Legend
- Treatment not recommended
+ Acceptable treatment
++ Optimal treatment

Figure 3.

Emphasis must again be placed on the importance of looking at the entire picture when characterizing a cartilage lesion. It is imperative to consider each lesion in the context of alignment, ligamentous and meniscal integrity, (Macroenvironment) as well as molecular level factors such as chondrocyte function, synovium, chondropenia and cartilage integrity, (Microenvironment). After completion of the comprehensive assessment described above, patients can then be stratified a clinical algorithm. This chondropenic pathway has been developed for the management of articular cartilage defects.

The algorithm defines ten patient-directed situations based on lesion size, depth, and associated issues such as alignment, ligament, and meniscal integrity. Each situation considers the problem category, the therapeutic options, and the current unresolved issues.

Situation No. 1
Problem: Meniscus tears and partial-thickness articular cartilage defect(s) (This is the most common condition the orthopaedic surgeon sees in practice).
Treatment Options: Arthroscopic debridement and partial meniscectomy followed by rehabilitation physical and conditioning therapy
Unresolved Issues: Role of radiofrequency probes. Do they cause chondrocyte death or decrease regenerative and more degenerative or avascular consequences (bipolar, monopolar)? Why and when to use of Glucosamine and Chrondroitin Sulfate and Viscosupplementation?

Situation No. 2
Problem: Femoral articular cartilage defects less than 1 cm^2.
Treatment Options: debridement, microfracture, osteochondral grafting
Unresolved Issues: Do small defects heal sufficiently well with mesenchymal stem-cell stimulation techniques such as microfracture in the short and long term?

Situation No. 3
Problem: Femoral articular cartilage defects including osteochondritis dissecans size 1 to 2 cm^2.
Therapeutic Primary Options: Debridement, microfracture, osteochondral grafting, autologous chondrocyte implantation
Therapeutic Secondary Options: Osteochondral grafting, autologous chondrocyte implantation
Unresolved Issues: Is a mesenchymal stem-cell stimulation technique an acceptable primary option?

Situation No. 4
Problem: Femoral articular cartilage defects including osteochondritis dissecans greater than 2 cm^2.
Therapeutic Primary Options: Autologous chondrocyte implantation, fresh allograft
Therapeutic Secondary Options: Autologous chondrocyte implantation, fresh allograft
Unresolved Issues: What is the optimal and maximal size of lesion that osteochondral autografts can be applied?

Situation No. 5
Problem: Complex femoral articular defects with malalignment, ligament, and/or meniscal deficiency.
Therapeutic Primary Options: Osteotomy, meniscal repair or allograft, cruciate reconstruction(s), autologous chondrocyte implantation, fresh allograft, or

osteochondral autograft depending on size

Unresolved Issues: How to optimally stage procedures so that index postoperative protocol does not compromise integrity of secondary or tertiary procedures. Which meniscus allograft, osteotomies, or ligament reconstruction procedure to utilize?

Situation No. 6

Problem: Patellar and/or trochlear articular cartilage defects with no malalignment or instability.

Therapeutic Primary Options: Physical and conditioning therapy including tapping bracing and pelvic stabilization.

Therapeutic Secondary Options: arthroscopy and lateral release, therapeutic tertiary options, autologous chondrocyte implantation plus anteromedialization or patellofemoral realignment osteotomy

Unresolved Issues: What are the definitive indications for arthroscopic lateral release? Does viscosupplementation have a role early in management of patellofemoral chondromalacia syndrome?

Situation No. 7

Problem: Patellar and trochlear articular cartilage defects, with significant malalignment, or instability.

Therapeutic Primary Options: Physical and conditioning therapy including tapping bracing and pelvic stabilization

Therapeutic Secondary Options: Autologous chondrocyte implantation plus anteromedialization or patellofemoral realignment osteotomy

Unresolved Issues: Is the role of osteotomy beneficial early on to disease modifying such that it will prevent OA of the patellofemoral joint?

Situation No. 8

Problem: Tibial articular cartilage defects--no significant malalignment or instability.

Therapeutic Options: Osteotomy as required in relation to the degree of malalignment in combination with microfracture or autologous chondrocyte implantation depending on size of lesion.

Unresolved Issues: Successful access may require release of collateral ligaments and detached meniscus insertions. Concomitant procedures protocols should not conflict with postoperative rehabilitative protocol.

Situation No. 9

Problem: Significant chondropenia and early OA (global Grade III/IV articular cartilage defects in the thirty- to sixty-year-old patient with degenerative meniscal tears).

Therapeutic Options: Nonsteroidal anti-inflammatory medications/Cox-2 inhibitors, hyaluronic acid, glucosamine/chondroitin sulfate, bike for exercise, unloading braces, arthroscopy for mechanical symptoms, loose bodies and meniscal tears, osteotomy selectively as required in relation to the degree of malalignment and/or joint-space narrowing.

Unresolved Issues: Is there a role for biological resurfacing procedures concomitant with realignment procedures?

Situation No. 10

Problem: Degenerative meniscal tears and global Grade IV defects (late OA).
Therapeutic Options: Nonsteroidal anti-inflammatory medications/Cox-2 inhibitors, hyaluronic acid, glucosamine/chondroitin sulfate, bike for exercise, unloading braces, arthroscopy for mechanical symptoms, loose bodies and meniscal tears, osteotomy selectively as required in relation to the degree of malalignment and/or joint-space narrowing, total knee arthroplasty.
Unresolved Issues: What is the role of arthroscopy in late OA other than alleviation of mechanical symptoms?

Conclusions and challenges

The challenges of articular cartilage repair and restoration continue despite recent advances. Marrow stimulation techniques, substitution replacement options and biologic replacement options each have a role in the treatment algorithm of articular cartilage defects. This treatment algorithim must take into account not only the characterization of the specific cartilage lesion but also the myriad of local and regional factors as well as the co-morbidities attached to each patient. As of yet no single treatment option can reestablish the hyaline cartilage seen in normal articular cartilage. The goal for future treatments is to develop new technologies and disease-modifying interventions that protect and preserve the joint over time by maintaining biochemical, biomechanical, and cellular integrity. Until these technologies exist, collaboration between the basic scientist and the clinician will continue to advance our current technologies in an effort to restore the violated articular cartilage surface.

References

1. Mithoefer K, McAdams TR, Scopp JM, Mandelbaum BR. Emerging options for treatment of articular cartilage injury in the athlete. Clin Sports Med. 2009 Jan;28(1):25-40.
2. Brittberg M, Peterson L, Sjögren-Jansson E, Tallheden T, Lindahl A. Articular cartilage engineering with autologous chondrocyte transplantation: a review of recent developments. J Bone Joint Surg Am. 2003;85(suppl 3):109-115.
3. Steadman JR, Briggs KK, Rodrigo JJ, Kocher MS, Gill TJ, Rodkey WG. Outcomes of microfracture for traumatic chondral defects of the knee: average 11-year follow-up. Arthroscopy. 2003;19:477-484.
4. Kon E, Delcogliano M, Filardo G, Montaperto C, Marcacci M. Second generation issues in cartilage repair. Sports Med Arthrosc. 2008 Dec;16(4):221-9. Review.
5. Buckwalter JA, Mankin HJ, Grodzinsky AJ. Articular cartilage and osteoarthritis. Instr Course Lect. 2005;54:465-80. Review.
6. Peterson L, Minas T, Brittberg M, Lindahl A. Treatment of osteochondritis dissecans of the knee with autologous chondrocyte transplantation: results at two to ten years. J Bone Joint Surg Am. 2003;85-A Suppl 2:17-24
7. Alford JW, Cole BJ. Cartilage restoration, part 1: basic science, historical perspective, patient evaluation, and treatment options. Am J Sports Med. 2005 Feb;33(2):295-306. Review.
8. Alford JW, Cole BJ. Cartilage restoration, part 2: techniques, outcomes, and future directions. Am J

Sports Med. 2005 Mar;33(3):443-60. Review

9. Potter HG, Black BR, Chong le R. New techniques in articular cartilage imaging. Clin Sports Med. 2009 Jan;28(1):77-94

10. Welsch GH, Mamisch TC, Quirbach S, Zak L, Marlovits S, Trattnig S. Evaluation and comparison of cartilage repair tissue of the patella and medial femoral condyle by using morphological MRI and biochemical zonal T2 mapping. Eur Radiol. 2008 Dec 23 [Epub ahead of print].

11. Outerbridge RE. The etiology of chondromalacia patellae. J Bone Joint Surg Br. 1961;43:752-759.

12. Insall J. Patellar pain. J Bone Joint Surg Am. 1982;64:147-152.

13. Bauer M, Jackson RW. Chondral lesions of the femoral condyles: a system of arthroscopic classification. Arthroscopy. 1988;4:97-102.

14. Noyes FR, Bassett RW, Grood ES, Butler DL. Arthroscopy in acute traumatic hemarthrosis of the knee: incidence of anterior cruciate tears and other injuries. J Bone Joint Surg Am. 1980;62:687-695,757.

15. International Cartilage Repair Society. The cartilage standard evaluation form/knee. ICRS Newsletter. 1998;1:5-7.

"Before anything else, preparation is the key to success"

(Alexander Graham Bell (1847-1922))

Chapter 9.

Debridement of Cartilage Lesions

Matej Drobnič

> **Take Home Message**
>
> • *A chronic cartilage lesion has a crater-like shape with osseous sclerosis in its base; it may be filled with degenerated cartilage and fibrotic tissue.*
> • *Cartilage lesion debridement by itself does not restore the cartilage, but it may offer temporary relief when small lesions with predominately mechanical symptoms are treated.*
> • *The role of the debridement combined with cell-based cartilage repair is to create a cleared contained lesion for the graft implantation.*
> • *The depth level of the debridement is defined by the technology for cell seeding used.*

Structure of a cartilage lesion

A histological section of a normal articular surface in adults reveals four cartilage zones (superficial, intermediate, deep, and calcified) that continue further into the subchondral endplate. A single continuous basophilic line "tide-mark" typically delineates deep and calcified zones in healthy and skeletally mature joints. In immature individuals the calcified zone is not formed yet, therefore the deep cartilage zone strongly interconnects with the subchondral endplate[1]. The lesion's natural history and also the recommendations for surgical interventions are defined by the lesion depth: partial thickness (ICRS Grades I or II), full thickness (ICRS Grade III), and osteochondral lesions (ICRS Grade IV) (Figure 1)[2].

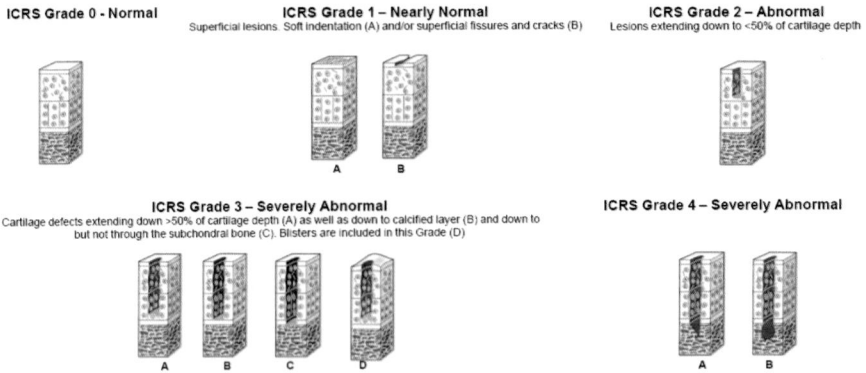

Images reproduced with authorization from the International Cartilage Repair Society - ICRS

Figure 1: ICRS criteria for grading of chondral lesions (2). Grades 1 and 2 represent partial thickness chondral lesions, grade 3 full thickness chondral lesions, and grade 4 osteochondral lesions.

Vertical walls and U-shape form of a lesion may be encountered acutely after the injury, however a typical chronic (osteo)chondral lesion has a cater-like appearance. There is slow depth progression from the uninjured margins toward the deepest central part. Parts of the chronic lesions, especially the ones with previously failed cartilage repair procedures, may be filled with degenerated cartilage, fibrosis, or mixture of both[3]. The calcified cartilage zone in such lesions is mostly abraded and the base of the lesion consists of sclerotic osseous tissue (Figure 2).

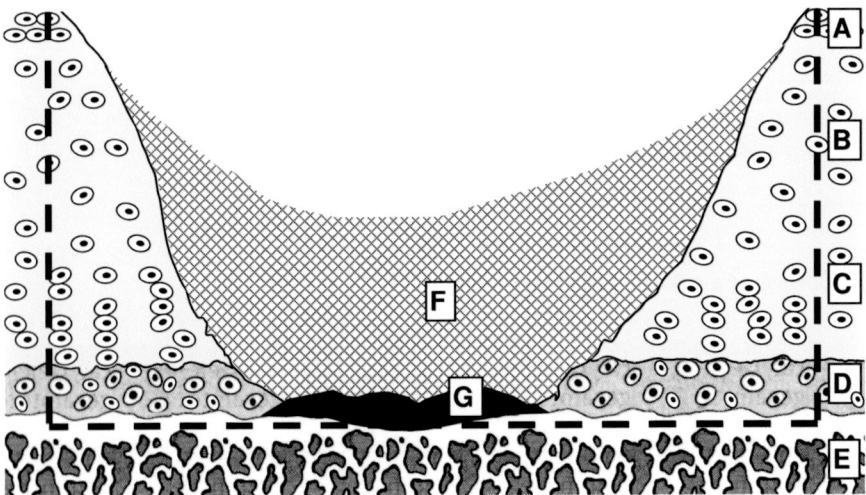

Figure 2: A schematic cross-section over a chronic full-thickness chondral lesion with a crater-like form. All cartilage layers (A – superficial, B – intermediate, C – deep, and D – calcified cartilage) are absent. A chronic lesion may be filled with a combination of degenerated cartilage and fibrous tissue (F); the base may consists of sclerotic bone invading the chondral layers (G). Dotted lines represent borders of an adequate lesion debridement prior to cell-based cartilage repair.

Lesion debridement as an isolated operative procedure

The open debridement for an osteoarthritic (OA) joint was popularized by Magnusson more than 60 years ago, but in the arthroscopic era this technique became widely accepted as the mainstay therapy for symptomatic joints with mild to moderate OA[4]. The goal of the procedure is mechanical removal of cartilage flaps and major fibrillations; non-aggressive shavers are typically used. The usage of radiofrequency chondroplasty for OA remains contradictory: the majority of ex-vivo studies demonstrated a detrimental effect of the RF probes on the chondrocyte viability[5], but the clinical studies favor their outcome in comparison to mechanical shaving[6]. However, due to recent studies with high medical evidence the clinical interest for the debridement of OA joints has been declining gradually. Their authors showed that arthroscopy for a degenerated knee provides no additional benefit to optimized physical and medical therapy[7,8].

The usage of cartilage debridement as an isolated procedure remains widely accepted for symptomatic isolated chondral lesions smaller than 2 cm^2 in less active patients[9]. The mechanical removal of unstable injured cartilage by various arthroscopic instruments (probes, graspers, curettes, or shavers) is quick, easy, inexpensive, and requires only a short rehabilitation. The isolated debridement is a purely palliative procedure that does not lead to the cartilage restoration in the lesion, but it may successfully target the mechanical symptoms, such as clicking or catching. Since the origin of cartilage-related pain is not well understood its reduction after the lesion debridement is unpredictable. The natural history of debrided small cartilage lesions remains unclear[10,11].

Lesion debridement prior to the cartilage repair

This cartilage lesion debridement is the first step of every cartilage repair procedure. The goal of the debridement is to create a contained (osteo)chondral lesion by removing any non-healthy tissue (degenerated cartilage, fibrosis, sclerotic bone). The lateral walls of a debrided lesion should be vertical and they should consist of healthy cartilage to ensure appropriate graft shouldering and secure attachment of marginal sutures for periosteum or membrane, in case they are needed[12]. The adequate technique of the debridement is particularly important for cell-based cartilage repair: classical or scaffold autologous chondrocyte implantation, bone marrow stimulation, injection of bone marrow aspirate, mesenchymal stem cells seeding, and others. An equine study on microfractures demonstrated improved repair tissue in the absence of calcified layer[13], but the most appropriate depth for the lesion debridement prior to the other cell-based techniques is not known. In general, an inadequate debridement generates a non-shouldered partial-thickness chondral lesion, with lateral walls of degenerated cartilage, while the excessive performance results in the subchondral endplate abrasion and in the unnecessary injury to the adjoining cartilage.

The osteochondral autografts and allografts typically anchor deep into the bone and the debridement is performed automatically by the recipient area preparation[14]. Same is true also for the novel cell-free scaffolds which rely on stem-cell inflow from the subchondral bone[15].

Debridement with the classical and scaffold autologous chondrocyte implantation (ACI)

According to the classical ACI method the subchondral endplate should not be violated to prevent from stem cells introduction with bleeding. In reality some minor bleeds from the subchondral base do occur and they are managed by pointed electro-cauterization or by local application of epinephrine, fibrin sealant, or haemostatic sponges. A bone grafting and a sandwich ACI technique is recommended when preceding procedures extensively damaged the subchondral endplate or if a primary osteochondral lesion deeper than 7–8 mm is encountered[16]. The debridement combined with classical ACI is typically performed openly by a scalpel (to define the lesion wall with the cut down to the bone) and a curette or raspatorium (to scrape away the tissue), which also demonstrated the most reliable performance in an ex-vivo study[17]. The surgeons typically rely on the basic subjective criteria when the debridement is completed: all the non-glassy or yellowish tissue down to the bone and laterally to the normal cartilage is removed, and no bleeding from the lesion base upon a tourniquet release is observed[12,16].

The debridement in combination with scaffold chondrocyte seeding is depending upon the strategy of the graft delivery: cutting out the graft according to the lesion size or covering the lesion with the pre-sized grafts in the mosaic manner. In the first cases the debridement follows rules of classical ACI technique, except that the arthroscopic manual curette is used[18,19]. When the pre-sized grafts are used, the debridement is conducted with special drills or abraders that fit the graft[20,21]. They can be introduced over a guide-wire or a guide-tube and have a safety stop at a designated depth. They typically abrade into the subchondral area to ensure a better graft stability and to remove the diseased bone. As the chondrocytes are incorporated in the scaffold biomaterial, the quality of repair tissue is supposed not to be compromised by the blood inflow.

Conclusions

The cartilage lesion debridement is and will remain the first step of every cartilage repair procedure. The usage of debridement as an isolated procedure should be limited to the patients with small lesion with predominately mechanical joint symptoms. The depth of the lesion debridement in the central part is mostly dictated by the cell scaffold used, but in the lateral walls the debridement has to reach the macroscopically normal cartilage.

References

1. Buckwalter JA; Mankin HJ, Articular cartilage: tissue design and chondrocyte-matrix interactions, Instr Course Lect, 1998, 47: 477-486
2. ICRS General Committee, ICRS Cartilage Injury Evaluation Package, http://www.cartilage. org/files/ICRS_evaluation.pdf, 2000
3. Drobnič M; Stražar K; Zupanc O; Cör A, Histology of chondral lesions before and after the classical debridement in patients appointed for the matrix-ACI, Abstract book of the 8th World Congress of ICRS, ICRS Miami, 2009, 176
4. Johnson LL, Arthroscopic abrasion arthroplasty: a review, Clin Orthop, 2001, 391 Suppl: 306-317
5. Caffey S; McPherson E; Moore B; Hedman T; Vangsness CT Jr, Effects of radiofrequency energy on human articular cartilage: an analysis of 5 systems, Am J Sports Med, 2005, 33: 1035-1039
6. Spahn G; Kahl E; Muckley T; Hofmann GO; Klinger HM, Arthroscopic knee chondroplasty using a bipolar radiofrequency-based device compared to mechanical shaver: results of a prospective, randomized, controlled study, Knee Surg Sports Traumatol Arthrosc, 2008, 16: 565-573
7. Kirkley A; Birmingham TB; Litchfield RB; Giffin JR; Willits KR; Wong CJ; Feagan BG; Donner A; Griffin SH; D'Ascanio LM; Pope JE; Fowler PJ, A randomized trial of arthroscopic surgery for osteoarthritis of the knee, N Engl J Med, 2008, 359: 1097-1107
8. Moseley JB; O'Malley K; Petersen NJ; Menke TJ; Brody BA; Kuykendall DH; Hollingsworth JC; Ashton CM; Wray NP, A controlled trial of arthroscopic surgery for osteoarthritis of the knee. N Engl J Med, 2002, 347: 81-88
9. Alford JW; Cole BJ, Cartilage restoration, part 2: techniques, outcomes, and future directions, Am J Sports Med, 2005, 33: 443-460
10. Fu FH; Zurakowski D; Browne JE; Mandelbaum B; Erggelet C; Moseley JB; Anderson AF; Micheli LJ, Autologous chondrocyte implantation versus debridement for treatment of full-thickness chondral defects of the knee: an observational cohort study with 3-year follow-up, Am J Sports Med 33, 2005: 1658-1666
11. Shelbourne KD; Jari S; Gray T, Outcome of untreated traumatic articular cartilage defects of the knee: a natural history study, J Bone Joint Surg Am, 2003, 85A Suppl 2: 8-16
12. Minas T; Peterson, Advanced techniques in autologous chondrocyte transplantation, Clin Sports Med, 1999, 18: 13-44
13. Frisbie DD; Morisset S; Ho CP; Rodkey WG; Steadman JR; McIlwraith CW, Effects of calcified cartilage on healing of chondral defects treated with microfracture in horses, Am J Sports Med, 2006, 34: 1824-1831
14. Hangody L; Feczko P; Bartha L; Bodo G; Kish G, Mosaicplasty for the treatment of articular defects of the knee and ankle, Clin Orthop, 2001, Suppl 391: 328-336
15. Williams RJ 3rd; Gamradt SC, Articular cartilage repair using a resorbable matrix scaffold. Instr Course Lect, 2008, 57: 563-571
16. Peterson L, International experience with autologous chondrocyte transplantation. In: Scott WN (ed), Insall & Scott Surgery of the Knee, 4th ed. Churchill Livingstone Elsevier, Philadelphia, 2006, 367–379
17. Drobnič M; Radosavljevič D; Cör A; Brittberg M; Stražar K, Debridement of cartilage lesions before autologous chondrocyte implantation by open or transarthroscopic techniques. A comparative study using post-mortem materials, J Bone Joint Surg Br, 2010, 92B: 602-608.
18. Erggelet C; Sittinger M; Lahm A, The arthroscopic implantation of autologous chondrocytes for the treatment of full-thickness cartilage defects of the knee joint, Arthroscopy, 2003, 19: 108-110

19. Ronga M; Grassi FA; Bulgheroni P, Arthroscopic autologous chondrocyte implantation for the treatment of a chondral defect in the tibial plateau of the knee, Arthroscopy, 2004, 20: 79-84

20. Ait Si Selmi T; Verdonk P; Chambat P; Dubrana F; Potel JF; Barnouin L; Neyret P, Autologous chondrocyte implantation in a novel alginate-agarose hydrogel: outcome at two years, J Bone Joint Surg Br, 2008, 90B: 597-604

21. Marcacci M; Kon E; Zaffagnini S; Filardo G; Delcogliano M; Neri MP; Iacono F, Hollander AP, Arthroscopic second generation autologous chondrocyte implantation, Knee Surg Sports Traumatol Arthrosc, 2007, 15: 610-619

"Symptoms are the body's mother tongue; signs are in a foreign language"

(John Brown)

Chapter 10.

The Treatment of Large Degenerative Defects

Stefano Zaffagnini, Giuseppe Filardo, Elizaveta Kon, Viviana Zarbà, Giulio Maria Marcheggiani Muccioli, Marco Delcogliano, Giovanni Giordano, Giovanni Ravazzolo, Maurilio Marcacci

Take Home Message

In the management of large cartilage lesions the treatment algorithm, usually used for small-medium defects, can not be easily applied.
Most of the numerous methods successfully proposed to restore the chondral surface offer good results especially in case of medium lesions in the young active population, whereas large degenerative pathology is still plagued by lower clinical outcome and a higher failure rate.
For large defects there is hope of future use of the rapidly growing knowledge on bioengineering and the development of new osteochondral scaffolds or cytokine-matrix metalloproteinase inhibitors.

Introduction

Degenerative articular cartilage lesions are difficult to treat and present a great challenge for orthopedic surgeons, due to the distinctive structure and function of hyaline cartilage, its inherent low healing potential and the numerous unknown factors that cause degeneration of the articular joint. The ultrastructure of articular cartilage is unique: chondrocytes are sparsely distributed within the surrounding matrix, maintaining minimal cell to cell contact. The interaction between cells, collagen framework, aggrecan and fluid constitute the complex biomechanical feature of hyaline cartilage making it difficult to repair, especially for large degenerative lesions. Biomechanical, metabolic and biological changes may led to the loss of tissue homeostasis, resulting in accelerated loss of articular surface and leading to end-stage arthritis. Moreover, the regeneration capacity of cartilage is limited due to its isolation from systemic regulation and its lack of vessels and nerve supply. None of the inflammatory processes is available for its repair and chondrocytes cannot migrate to the site of injury from an intact healthy site, unlike most tissue. In fact, even small isolated injuries to the cartilage of the knee are difficult to heal and represent a risk factor for further degeneration, leading to more extensive joint damage, in relation to higher mechanical stress on the lesion's edge[1,2,3].

Unfortunately, the incidence of articular cartilage lesions has grown, due to the marked increase in sports participation and greater emphasis on physical activity in all age groups, and the expectations of patients about recovery have raisen as well. Curl[4] found a 63% incidence of chondral lesion in a survey of 31,516 knee arthroscopies, and joint degeneration has become the most common joint disorder in developed countries. An increased prevalence of osteoarthritis has also been documented: from 1995 to 2005 the number people affected with symptomatic OA has grown from 21 million to nearly 27 million in the United States[5]. Pain from joint degeneration is a key symptom in the decision to seek medical care and is an important antecedent to disability. The rapid increase in the prevalence of this already common disease explains the growing impact on health care and public health systems. For these reasons, in recent years orthopaedic surgeons have tried to identify an efficient treatment for full thickness articular surface lesions of the knee. Currently, different approaches have been proposed to treat this pathology and numerous therapeutic options have been used for the treatment of cartilage lesions with variable success rates.

Treatments

Numerous agents, such as nonsteroidal anti-inflammatory drugs, glucosamine, chondroitin sulfate, hyaluronic acid and glucocorticoids have been proposed as non invasive solution for pain treatment, improvement in function and disability, and ultimately modification of chondral lesions and osteoarthritis. An initial pharmacologic management typically begins with analgesia and anti-inflammatory agents, through acetaminophen and NSAIDs. However, the potential cardiovascular and gastrointestinal toxicity, the large apparent variation in individual response to each drug and the absence of clear clinical data regarding the therapeutic potentiality represent the major limits of this therapeutic approach. Topical agents, used as adjuncts or in patients in whom systemic medications are problematic, have only been proven useful for short-term use of mild to moderate pain in no severe chondropathies[6]. Intra-articular injections of corticosteroids, such as few studies indicate, are of short-term benefit for pain and function[7]. Moreover, some evidence suggests that they are not able to alter the natural history of the disease and may also have deleterious consequences on knee structures. Glucosamine, chondroitin and intra-articular hyaluronic acid have not been clearly demonstrated to be effective[8,9], too, and due to the continuing controversies and lack of common accepted beneficial evidence should not be considered ideal procedures for the treatment of chondropathies. Researcher are therefore investigating new methods of stimulating repair or replacing damaged cartilage, such as matrix metalloproteinase inhibitors, gene therapy, cytokine inhibitors, artificial cartilage substitutes and growth factors[10]. Laboratory investigations are focusing on the possibility of preserving normal homeostasis or blocking or reversing structural damage as a target, in order to avoid or at least delay the need of more invasive surgical procedures. Current pharmacological interventions may temporarily reduce chronic pain but at the time being no proven disease-modifying therapy is available.

Temporary bracing, radiation, magnetic field[11] and physiotherapy are also initially applied as conservative treatments but, in most of the cases, large cartilage defects require a more invasive treatment with a surgical approach, in order to restore the chondral articular surface.

Various techniques, both reparative and regenerative, have been used to treat this pathology. Treatment options directed to the recruitment of bone marrow cells to obtain potential cartilage precursors have been developed to allow stem cells migration from the marrow cavity to the fibrin clot of the defect. Steadman[12] has reported satisfactory results at 11 years follow-up with microfracture technique; however, patients may have to adjust their activity level to that of their knee function. Microfracture technique is simple and can be used in small lesions or in selected cases in wide degenerative lesions. However, the repair tissue response can be unpredictable; fibrous soft, spongiform tissue combined with central degeneration is frequently founded, and the clinical failure has been observed at a mean time of 21 months after treatment[13]. In fact, these treatment options, such as abrasion, drilling and microfracture, produce predominantly a fibrous repair tissue, with mostly type I collagen fibrocytes and an unorganized matrix, which lacks the biomechanical and viscoelastic characteristics of normal hyaline cartilage. Recent literature[14] has also shown that these techniques can be used with less favourable outcome in large defects even if they are appealing to the surgeon because they are single–stage procedures, cost effective and with minimal morbidity. The results showed in the literature[15] suggest to reserve these procedures for the treatment of acute and small lesions, whereas they are not indicated in case of large cartilage defects.

Another approach for repairing large osteochondral lesions is represented by reconstructive surgical treatments, such as osteochondral autograft transfer and mosaicplasty[16]. This procedures guarantee an immediate reliable tissue transfer of viable osteochondral units and aim to capitalize on bone-to-bone healing, since the mature cartilaginous tissue has limited healing potential and heals completely with difficulty to surrounding cartilage. An autologous osteochondral graft can be applied by arthroscopic or open surgery, depending on size and site of the articular defect, with low surgical and post-surgical stress for the patients, and this method seems to be the only surgical technique capable of immediately restoring the height and shape of an articular surface in focal osteochondral defects in one surgical step. Good results from this technique are

reported in the literature: Hangody[16] evaluated the clinical outcome of 831 patients who underwent mosaicplasty and reported 92% good-to-excellent clinical results in case of femoral condylar implants, and a comparative prospective
evaluation of 413 arthroscopic resurfacing procedures (mosaicplasty, drilling,
abrasion and microfractures) showed that mosaicplasty gave a more favourable
clinical outcome in the long-term follow-up[17]. We[18] found satisfactory results at
2 and 7 years' follow-up in small (not more than 2-5 cm^2) grade III-IV lesions of
femoral condyles in young and middle-aged patients with no significant clinical
worsening, showing the persistence of the results if the technique is used with
correct indications. We observed that the number of plugs significantly inversely
affects the clinical outcome. A high number of grafts can promote the formation of a large amount of fibrous tissue filling the space between the plugs and
also increase the incidence of technical problems, compromising the mechanical properties of the reconstructed zone. It is also difficult to obtain the physiological curvature of an articular surface, this could produce an abnormal stress
distribution and subsequent suffering of the implant. Furthermore, the stability
of the plug in the subchondral bone can be weaker due to excessive reaming.
The procedure is therefore technically demanding and the complete coverage
of the defect, especially for large lesions, is critical. Graft availability is another
important issue, which severely reduces the possibility of using these procedures
for the treatment of large defects. We have published[19] a series of large massive
osteochondral unit implant performed with open surgery. The graft is harvested
with scalpels of different length from the medial superior area of the grove and
inserted press fit in the condylar defect previously prepared. The results at 5 years
were good in 92% of the patients, with complete restoration of the articular surface (Fig. 1,2).

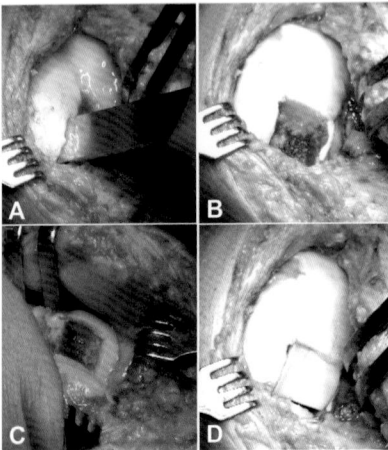

Figure 1: Large cartilage lesion (A) of the femoral condyle. The defect is prepared (B) and filled with a massive osteochondral unit (D) harvested from a non-weight-bearing area (C).

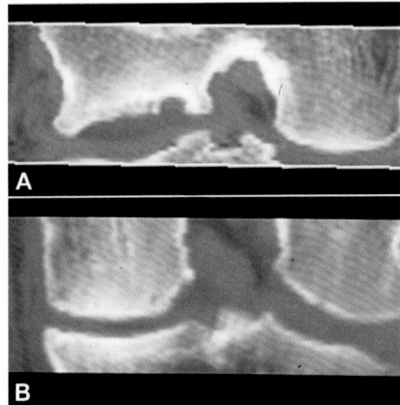

Figure 2: Preoperative and 6 years follow up TC images of a large femoral condyle lesion treated with a massive osteochondral autologous graft.

In the really large defects, a valid alternative option is the use of homologous osteochondral grafts. The easy management of stored osteochondral allografts allows to use them as scaffold with high biomechanical properties and low antigenicity for the treatment of big articular lesions. However, stored grafts don't maintain their biological and biomechanical characteristics, with loss of chondrocytes vitality and worsening of biomechanical properties[20,21]. On the contrary, fresh osteochondral allografts preserve tissue vitality and offer good long term results with graft survival and satisfactory clinical outcome[22]. Unfortunately, despite this procedure has been successfully used for the treatment of large chondral defects, there are still some concerns. The low availability and the difficulties in the preservation and management of the fresh allografts and the increased risk of disease transmission reduce the indication and the wider use of this technically demanding procedure. In fact, we reserve the use of this surgical approach only for the treatment of massive osteochondral lesions in young patients with high functional requirements, otherwise doomed to poor clinical outcome, in order to avoid or at least delay the need of knee arthroplasty (Fig. 3).

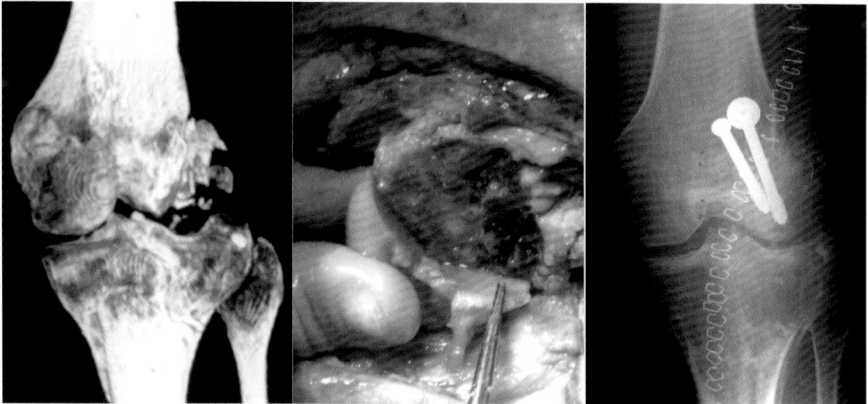

Figure 3: Massive osteochondral lesion of the lateral femoral condyle treated with a fresh allograft.

Given the intrinsic limitations of these techniques, in recent years newer surgical approaches have been proposed to replace cartilage defects with newly grown mature cartilage. Regenerative techniques, such as autologous chondrocyte implantation (ACI), have been developed and have emerged as a potential therapeutic option aimed at restoring a completely normal joint.

Since being introduced in Sweden in 1987, the cell-based approach has gained increasing acceptance and recent studies highlight the long-term durable nature of this form of treatment, due to the production of hyaline-like cartilage that is mechanically and functionally stable and integrates into the adjacent articular surface[23]. However, these good results have to be weighed against the number of problems that can be observed with the standard ACI methods. First generation ACI has been associated with several limitations related to the complexity and morbidity of the surgical procedure. This technique requires a large joint exposure with a high risk of joint stiffness and arthrofibrosis. Moreover, there is a frequent occurrence of periosteal hypertrophy, that often requires revision surgery. At these problems simply related to the surgical procedure we must add the technical problems of the culture and transplantation procedure, such as maintenance of chondrocyte phenotype, non homogeneous cell distribution in the three dimensional spaces of the defect and cell loss using liquid suspension. Taking into consideration all these factors, a new generation procedure for cartilage transplantation was developed. The so-called second generation ACI technique uses a new tissue-engineering technology to create a cartilage-like tissue in a three-dimensional culture system with the attempt to address all the concerns related to the cell culture and the surgical technique. Essentially, the concept is based on the use of biodegradable polymers as temporary scaffolds for the in vitro growth of living cells and their subsequent transplantation onto the defect site. Various synthetic or natural materials in a variety of physical forms (fibers, meshes, gels), such as hyaluronan, collagen, fibrin glue, alginate, agarose and polylactides, were developed during last years and applied to cartilage tissue engineering[24]. On the basis of published results, the matrix-assisted chondrocyte implantation guarantees results comparable, even better of the traditional ACI technique, and simplifies the procedure with marked advantages from a biological and surgical point of view. Furthermore, the easy handling of some of the scaffolds allowed to develop arthroscopic implantation techniques[25]. Results of this new bioengineered approach are promising, but there is no agreement about the effective superiority of the cellular based procedures relative to others[26]. We compared[27] arthroscopic second generation autologous chondrocyte implantation on hyaluronic acid based scaffolds with microfracturing, and we obtained satisfactory clinical outcome in both groups of patients. However, whereas the results were comparable at 2 years follow up, more durable good clinical results and sport activity resumption were founded in the group treated with second generation ACI at further follow-up, as assessed by the 5 years evaluation.

The results of these techniques at medium term follow-up for the treatment of small-medium cartilage lesions have been documented and are satisfactory[24]. On the other hand, it has to be emphasized that treatment of large chondral pathology is controversial and presently none of existing first and second generation autologous chondrocytes products are indicated in generalized degenerative joint disease, yet. In fact, prospective studies on this type of patients are difficult to perform because cartilage defects are usually combined with malalignment of the lower limb or postmeniscectomy patients, and associated pathology should be addressed in order to possibly improve the clinical outcome. Therefore, it is difficult to evaluate the effectiveness of ACI in these combined pathologies.

The possibility to treat early stage arthritic lesions with tissue engineered cartilage is very attractive. However, it has to be kept in mind that in large cartilage lesions the subchondral bone is involved in the degenerative process, too. The treatment of osteo-cartilaginous unit is more problematic, because tissue damage involves two different tissues characterized by different intrinsic healing capacity. Tissue engineering techniques generally aim to regenerate only cartilage tissue and in case of osteochondral damage additional autologous bone grafting is often necessary. In case of large defects, biphasic scaffolds are preferable (Fig. 4), to reproduce the different biological and functional requirements for guiding the growth of the two tissues with a simple one-stage procedure. Moreover, as already underlined, co-morbidity like meniscal damage, ligament laxity or mechanical malalignment of the tibio-femoral or patello-femoral joint, are often associated to wide cartilage pathology and must be corrected before or at the same time that we treat the cartilage defect. In fact, instability or mechanical overloading of affected knee compartment, due to meniscal lack or misalignment, may jeopardize the graft and compromise the final outcome.

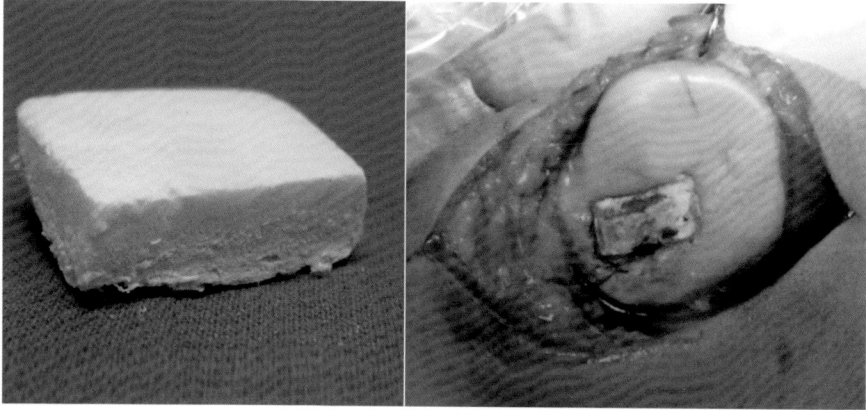

Figure 4: Treatment of a patellar lesion with a biphasic osteochondral scaffold.

The goals of the treatment consist on restoring the articular surface as much as possible obtaining a pain-free range of motion and the full recover of the previous activity level, and correct all the co-morbidity that may contribute to the joint pathology and impede the tissue regeneration. Treatments like osteotomy, ACL or peripheral structures reconstruction and meniscus allograft transplant are often required. For wide complex lesions, a distractor external fixator can be also applied in order to increase the joint stability and avoid compressive forces on the articular surface in the early maturation process of cartilage regeneration, especially when kissing lesions are present. We developed a new hinged dynamic external distractor, which allows to protect the graft and at the same time permits an immediate and safe postoperative joint mobilization with partial weight bearing and faster functional recovery[28] (Fig. 5).

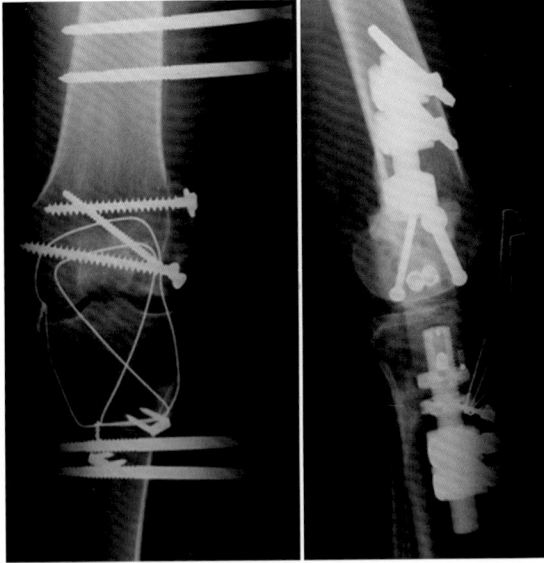

Figure 5: X Ray: application of a new hinged dynamic external distractor to protect an osteochondral allograft of the lateral femoral condyle.

In conclusion, the management of large cartilage lesions is challenging. Summing up, the treatment of this pathology is difficult and a single treatment modality may not be sufficient. A complex approach, involving multiple biological and biomechanical treatments, is often needed, and a long adequate rehabilitation program is also crucial to optimize the results of surgery improving the cartilage maturation process. Only a multifactorial approach with combined procedures could avoid or at least delay further joint degeneration and the need of more invasive and sacrificing procedures like TKA.

Conclusions

In the management of large cartilage lesions the treatment algorithm, usually used for small-medium defects, can not be easily applied. Most of the numerous methods successfully proposed to restore the chondral surface offer good results especially in case of medium lesions in the young active population, whereas large degenerative pathology is still plagued by lower clinical outcome and a higher failure rate. Several improvements are soon expected, as the result of the rapidly growing knowledge on bioengineering and the development of new osteochondral scaffolds or cytokine-matrix metalloproteinase inhibitors.
Studies on some new biomaterials are in progress, aiming to induce "in situ" regeneration after direct transplantation onto the defect site. The possibility to create a cell-free implant to be sufficiently "intelligent" to bring into the joint the appropriate cues to induce orderly and durable osteochondral regeneration in one step-surgery is very attractive and is under investigation.

The improvement in tissue engineering with development of new scaffolds and an integrated biological and biomechanical surgical approach may offer an interesting therapeutic option even for difficult cases with large cartilage defects and joint degeneration, otherwise doomed to poor results, leading to a more reliable and biological procedure and possibly better clinical outcome.

Acknowledgements

S. Bassini: IX Division – Biomechanic Lab, Rizzoli Orthopedic Institute, Bologna, Italy.

References

1. Buckwalter JA; Mankin HJ, Articular cartilage, J Bone Joint Surg, 1997, 79A (4): 600-611
2. Buckwalter JA; Mankin HJ, Articular cartilage. Part II: Degeneration and osteoarthrosis, repair, regeneration, and tranplantation, J Bone Joint Surg, 1997, 79A (4): 612-632
3. Wong B; Cigan A; Kim S; Sah R, The effect of a focal articular defetc on cartilage deformation during articulation, Proceedings of 55° Annual Meeting ORS, Las Vegas, Feb 22-25, 2009, Paper No. 149
4. Curl WW; Krome J; Gordon ES; Rushing J; Smith BP; Poehling GG, Cartilage injuries: a review of 31,516 knee arthroscopies, Arthroscopy, 1997, 13 (4): 456-460
5. Zhang Y; Jordan JM, Epidemiology of osteoarthritis, Rheum Dis Clin North Am, 2008, 34 (3): 515-529
6. Niethard FU; Gold MS; Solomon GS; et al, Efficacy of topical diclofenac diethylamine gel in osteoarthritis of the knee, J Reumatol, 2005, 32 (12): 2384-2392
7. Bellamy N; Campbell J; Robinson V; et al, Intra-articular corticosteroid for treatment of osteoarthritis of the knee, Cochrane Database Sys Rev, 2006, (2)
8. Reichenbach S; Trelle S; et al, Efficacy and safety of intra-articular hylan or hyaluronic acids for osteoarthritis of the knee: a randomized controlled trial, Arthritis Rheum, 2007, 56 (11): 3610-3619
9. Clegg DO; Reda DJ; Harris CL; et al, Glucosamine, Chondroityn sulfate, and the two in cambination for painful knee osteoarthritis, N Engl J Med, 2006, 354 (8): 795-808
10. Ulrich-Vinther M; Maloney MD; Schwarz EM; Rosier R; O'Keefe RJ, Articular cartilage biology, J Am Acad Orthop Surg, 2003, 11 (6): 421-430
11. Fini M; Giavaresi G; Torricelli P; Cavani F; Setti S; Canè V; Giardino R, Pulsed electromagnetic fields reduce knee osteoarthritic lesion progression in the aged Dunkin Hartley guinea pig, J Orthop Res, 2005, 23 (4): 899-908
12. Steadman JR; Briggs KK; Rodrigo JJ; Kocher MS; Gill TJ; Rodkey WG, Outcomes of microfracture for traumatic chondral defects of the knee: Average 11-year follow-up, Arthroscopy, 2003, 19 (5): 477-484
13. Nehrer S; Spector M; Minas T, Histologic analysis of tissue after failed cartilage repair procedures, Clin Orthop, 1999, 365: 149-162
14. Asik M; Ciftci F; Sen C; Erdil M; Atalar A, The microfracture technique for the treatment of full-thickness articular cartilage lesions of the knee: midterm results, Arthroscopy, 2008, 24 (11): 1214-1220
15. Williams RJ 3rd; Harnly HW, Microfracture: indications, technique, and results, Instr Course Lect, 2007; 56: 419-428
16. Hangody L; Fules P, Autologous osteochondral mosaicplasty for the treatment of full-thickness defects of weight-bearing joints, J Bone Joint Surg Am, 2003, 85 A (Suppl 2): 25-32
17. Hangody L; Feczkò P; Bartha L; Bodò G; Kish G, Mosaicplasty for the treatment of articular defects of the knee and ankle, Clin Orthop Rel Res, 2001, 391S: 326-336
18. Marcacci M; Kon E; Delcogliano M; Filardo G; Busacca M; Zaffagnini S, Arthroscopic autologous osteochondral grafting for cartilage defects of the knee: prospective study results at a minimum 7-year follow-up, Am J Sports Med, 2007, 35 (12): 2014-2021
19. Marcacci M; Kon E; Zaffagnini S; Visani A, Use of autologous grafts for reconstruction of osteochondral defects of the knee, Orthopedics, 1999, 22 (6): 595-600
20. Ohlendorf C; et al, Chondrocytes survival in cryopreserved osteochondral articulra cartilage, J Orthop Res, 1996, 14: 413-416

21. Pelker RR; et al, Biomechanical proprerties of bone allografts, Clin Orthop Relat Res, 1983, 174: 54-57

22. Gross AE; Shasha N; Aubin P, Long-term followup of the use of fresh osteochondral allografts for posttraumatic knee defects, Clin Orthop Relat Res, 2005, 435: 79-87

23. Peterson L; Brittberg M; Kiviranta I; Akerlund EL; Lindahl A, Autologous chondrocyte transplantation. Biomechanics and long-term durability, Am J Sports Med, 2002, 30 (1): 2-12

24. Kon E; Delcogliano M; Filardo G; Montaperto C; Marcacci M, Second generation issues in cartilage repair, Sports Med Arthrosc, 2008, 16 (4): 221-229

25. Marcacci M; Zaffagnini S; Kon E; Visani A; Iacono F; Loreti I, Arthroscopic autologous chondrocyte transplantation: technical note, Knee Surg Sports Traumatol Arthrosc, 2002, 10 (3): 154-159.

26. Knutsen G; Drogset JO; Engebretsen L; Grøntvedt T; Isaksen V; Ludvigsen TC; Roberts S; Solheim E; Strand T; Johansen O, A randomized trial comparing autologous chondrocyte implantation with microfracture. Findings at five years, J Bone Joint Surg Am, 2007, 89 (10): 2105-2112

27. Kon E; Gobbi A; Filardo G; Delcogliano M; Zaffagnini S; Marcacci M, Arthroscopic second-generation autologous chondrocyte implantation compared with microfracture for chondral lesions of the knee: prospective nonrandomized study at 5 years, Am J Sports Med, 2009, 37 (1): 33-41

28. Zaffagnini S; Iacono F; Lo Presti M; Di Martino A; Chochlidakis S; Elkin DJ; Giordano G; Marcacci M, A new hinged dynamic distractor, for immediate mobilization after knee dislocations: Technical note, Arch Orthop Trauma Surg, 2008, 128 (11): 1233-1237

"From the bitterness of disease man learns the sweetness of health"

(Catalan proverb)

CHAPTER 11.

UNLOADING OF THE REPAIRED CARTILAGE LESION. WHY, WHEN AND HOW

Mats Brittberg

Take Home Message

One has to protect the cartilage repair tissue if the defect area resurfaced is large even if there is no significant malalignment: use Unloader braces and/or Valgus or varus unloading osteotomy
• The position of the osteotomy is crucial-
• Remember the influence of the tibial slope on lesion site
• And equal when to treat patellar lesions with unloading tibial tubercle transfers
• An increased BMI (greater than 30) may have an adverse effect on some cartilage repair procedures.

Introduction

The chondrocyte is to be regarded as a cell under pressure. Mechanical load is an important regulator of the chondrocyte metabolic activity and subsequently cartilage proteoglucan content is highest in heavily loaded areas[11,13]
Cells in vitro could produce a cartilaginous layer however with a collagen layer about on half of native cartilage. The right type of collagen, type II, the major extracellular material that holds together tissues and organs of most complex organisms is needed. Weight bearing, may be a way to stimulate release of tran-

scription factors that could trigger a chondrocyte switch to produce the right amount and type of collagen. The degree of weight bearing after different cartilage repair methods has yet to be defined.

However, it has been reported that in the same patient a high loaded chondrocyte grafted area gives a more hyaline-like repair tissue compared to a less loaded chondrocyte grafted area that produced a more fibrocartilaginous repair[9].

Cartilage defects that have been nicely repaired with autologous chondrocyte implantation sometimes after some years deteriorate and more often in large defects, poorly contained lesions where a continuous high load may induce a PML, progressive matrix loss.

Similar with large defects treated by other cartilage repair methods. To protect cartilage repair with temporary or definite unloading of the treated area may seem important (Figs 1,2).

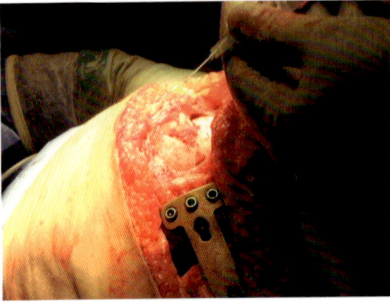

Figure 1: A large condylar cartilage defect treated by ACI (Hyalograft) glued to the defect + unloading with an opening wedge osteotomy with a Tomofix plate plate.

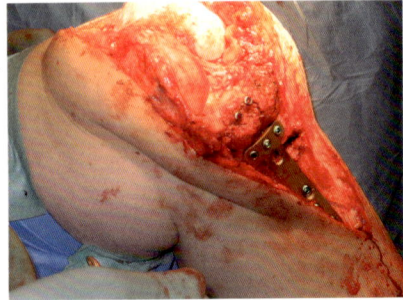

Figure 2: A large osteochondral defect of a tbial plateau treated by chondrocytes implantation in Hyalograft, + subchondral bone grafting followed by an unloading with an opening wedge osteotomy and Tomofix plate.

The main principle of osteotomies is to achieve a transfer of loading from diseased articular joint areas to areas with relatively intact, healthy cartilage

Different loading is depending on different cartilage lesions sizes and if the lesions are uni- or bi-polar lesions.

Guettler et al in 2004[5] showed that rim stress concentration becomes a factor for defects 10 mm in diameter (0.79 cm^2) and greater in size and that biomechanically, a "threshold effect" does indeed exist. This finding is in contrast to indications that a significant biomechanical alteration in local contact stress is appreciated at about 2 cm^2 (16-mm defect), which is most commonly quoted size in contemporary treatment algorithms. A threshold effect does occur at which rim stress concentration becomes a factor around osteochondral defects. Although the risk of lesion progression to arthritis is certainly multifactorial, rim stress concentration and altered loading may cause degeneration of adjacent cartilage[5].

When to perform an unloading

When the time is to do an unloading osteotomy will be depending on several factors such as lesion size, alignment, degree of Instability and body weight.

The unloading procedure may then be either a temporary unloading with an unloader brace or a definitive unloading with an unloading osteotomy.

The indications could be for large defects in a joint without any malalignment, small-large defects in a joint with malalignment and all defects with surrounding poor quality cartilage might be considered for unloading.

It is wise that in all investigations prior to surgery in patients with cartilage lesions, long weight bearing x-rays for measurement of HKA (Hip-Knee-Angle) are taken.

Scintigraphic examination to get a prognosis of the metabolic processes in the cartilage when cartilage lesions exist in a joint with degenerative cartilage could also be included when in doubt that an osteotomy is needed. A high uptake may indicate the risk of progress into OA and an indication to repair the local defect in combination with osteotomy.

The ideal correction method is to align the mechanical axis to pass through a point 30 to 40 percent lateral to the midpoint[3].

Studies about the effect of unloading local cartilage defects

Fujisawa et al.[3] have shown that if ideal correction was obtained, it was observed by arthroscopy that repair of the ulcerated region was initiated by the surviving cartilage in the affected area and the cartilage bordering the affected area.

Furthermore, the authors could also note that at about one and one-half to two years after osteotomy the ulcerated region was thoroughly covered with fibrous and membranous tissue[3].

Mina et al.[7] looked at high tibial osteotomies that was performed on 8 human cadaveric knees and was fixed with a dynamic external fixator. The fixator was used to vary the tibiofemoral alignment from 12° valgus to 10° varus.For all defect sizes, all contact pressure within the medial compartment was shifted to the lateral compartment at between 6° and 10° of valgus.

Contact pressure was found to concentrate around the defect rims for all defect sizes.

In addition, regarding the use of high tibial osteotomy for unloading isolated chondral defects,the authors found that contact pressure is approximately equally distributed between the medial and lateral compartments for alignments of 0° to 4° of valgus[7].

To avoid overloading the lateral compartment in patients with isolated chondral defects and varus malalignment, overcorrection to 8° to 10° of valgus is generally avoided[7].

Instead, most authors aim for correction to neutral or slightly valgus tibiofemoral alignments.

At between 0° and 4° of valgus, the authors found that contact pressure is approximately equally distributed between the medial and lateral compartments.

This loading situation most closely approximates physiologic loading and there-fore represents an ideal outcome for patients with isolated chondral defects[7].
Kanamiya et al.[6] studied osteotomies in 58 knees in 47 patients. The patients underwent a second look arthroscopic evaluation of the articular cartilage 18 months after surgery. Partial or even coverage with fibrocartilage (grade 3 and 4) was achieved on 55% of the femorotibial joint surfaces. A repair with white scat-tering with fibrocartilage (grade 2) was achieved in 34%, and 3 knees showed no regenerative change (grade 1)[6].
However, these results suggest that an adequate lateral deviation of the me-chanical axis promotes regeneration of the eburnated surface and that such an unloading could also be beneficial to a local cartilage repair process.
Specifically, satisfactory clinical results after HTO were seen in knees in which the mechanical axis passed within the lateral compartment (approximately 75%)[6].
Therefore, a proper correction after HTO is necessary to promote the regenera-tion of an eburnated surface.

Timing of the osteomy procedure

Cicuttini et al.[2] examined patients with asymptomatic knee cartilage defects identified by magnetic resonance imaging (MRI) and determined their rate of annual tibial cartilage volume loss during a 2-year period compared with a con-trol group. In patients with medial chondral defects, the annual rate of cartilage volume loss was 2.5%, compared with 1.3% in those patients without defects[2]. These natural history studies are the primary rationale for early intervention in symptomatic patients with focal articular damage of medium size to large le-sions.

My choices:
• Opening wedge ostetomies for medial lesions (Otis-plate, Tomifix-plate, Puddu plate)
• Opening wedge osteomies with Orthofix and callus distration for large mala lignments to correct
• Opening wedge osteotomies with Orthofix and callus distraction for lateral le sions less than 12 degrees of valgus

• **Controversial:**
• Look at both legs. Ex: The unaffected leg could be in 6 degrees varus. The affected lateral lesion knee in 1 degree varus. The osteotomy could aim to return that knee to 3-4 degree varus in order to unload enough for pain relief.

Supracondylar femoral varus osteotomy if the valgus deformity is more than 12 degrees of valgus or if the tilt of the tibial joint surface is more than 10 degrees.

Tibial slope
An opening wedge increases the posterior tibial slope ca 4 degrees.

An opening wedge has consequences on ACL insufficiency but also on where the cartilage lesion site is located[10].

A decrease of posterior tibial slope is recommended for: ACL-deficient and ACL-reconstructed knees and for isolated posterior femoral condyle and tibialplateau osteochondral defects recducing joint compression forces posteriorly[10]

An increase in tibial slope is desired for a PCL deficient knee, to treat PCL instability or to protect PCL reconstruction, isolated anterior cartilage lesions[10]

Lateral subluxation and tilt frequently leads to Patella OA

An abnormal lateral position of the tibial tuberosity causes distal malalignment of the extensor mechanism of the knee and can lead to lateral tracking of the patella causing anterior knee pain or objective patellar instability, characterised by recurrent dislocation[4].

Fulkerson Osteotomy[1,4]:
- modification of the Elmslie-Trillat Procedure, but involves anterior displacement as well;

- allows anteriorization of up to 15 mm, which should decrease lateral facet contact pressure;

• **Hauser Procedure:**
- involves medialization of the tibial tubercle inorder to decrease Q angle;
- due to the anatomy of the proximal tibia, translating the tibial tubercle medially, will also translate the tubercle posteriorly;
- posterior translation of the tibial tubercle will have the effect of increasing patellofemoral contact pressures which leads to DJD;
• As noted by Ferguson et al, elevation of 1.25 cm decreases patellofemoral contact forces by 60-80%4, but further elevation provided less benefit;
• usually no more than 1 cm of medialization is needed

Medialization may cause to much medial loading[4]. Be careful when to treat medial lesions!
Hauser plasty as it is a posteromedial transfer could cause medial patellar cartilage breakdown!!

• The patella will be articulating on more proximal cartilage with the knee flexed
• This lesion responds poorly to tibial tubercle anteriorization procedures as such an operation causes load shift onto more proximal patella

Re-routing osteotomies
• An overly medialized tibial tubercle with a painful and poorly repaired carti
lage patellar lesion may need to be returned to a lateral position via anterolateral tibial tubercle transfer[4].
• Lateral release will relieve abnormal tilt of the patella but if there is lateral facet
degeneration also osteotomy is needed.
• Anteromedial Tib.Tubercle transfer

Overweight

An increased BMI (greater than 30) may have an adverse effect on some cartilage
repair procedures[8]. Weight reducing is consequently an important part of all unloading protocols.

The future

Tissue engineering is an increasing research area. Future treatment of osteoarthritis and large osteochondral loss may be feasible. Unloading procedures will
be needed to unload the juvenile repair for the ultimate success (Figure 3).

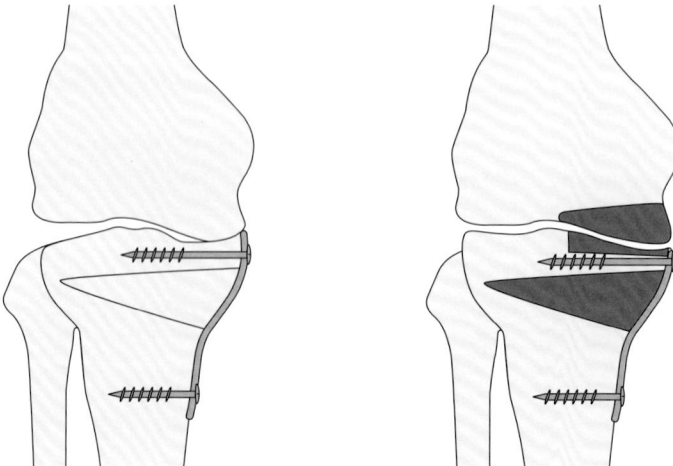

*Figure 3: Future tissue engineering. A grade III osteoarthritic lesion in a medial knee
compartment. Possible treatment is an opening wedge osteotomy to unload the
destroyed area + implantation of bipolar osteochondral cell-scaffold composites.*

References

1. Carofino BC, Fulkerson JP. Anteromedialization of the tibial tubercle for patellofemoral arthritis in
patients > 50 years.J Knee Surg. 2008 Apr;21(2):101-5
2.Cicuttini F, Ding C, Wluka A, Davis S, Ebeling PR, Jones G. Association of cartilage defects with loss of

knee cartilage in healthy, middle-age adults: a prospective study.Arthritis Rheum. 2005 Jul;52(7): 2033-9

3. Fujisawa Y, Masuhara K, Shiomi S. The effect of high tibial osteotomy on osteoarthritis of the knee. An arthroscopic study of 54 knee joints.Orthop Clin North Am. 1979 Jul;10(3):585-608.

4. Fulkerson JP.Articular cartilage lesions in patellofemoral pain patients. In Disorders of the patellofemoral joint. Fulkerson JP,Williams and Wilkins Baltimore 1997 p 225-274

5. Guettler JH, Demetropoulos CK, Yang KH, Jurist KA. Osteochondral defects in the human knee: influence of defect size on cartilage rim stress and load redistribution to surrounding cartilageAm J Sports Med. 2004 Sep;32(6):1451-8.

6. Kanamiya T, Naito M, Hara M, Yoshimura I. The influences of biomechanical factors on cartilage regeneration after high tibial osteotomy for knees with medial compartment osteoarthritis: clinical and arthroscopic observations.Arthroscopy. 2002 Sep;18(7):725-9

7. Mina C, Garrett WE Jr, Pietrobon R, Glisson R, Higgins L. High tibial osteotomy for unloading osteochondral defects in the medial compartment of the knee. Am J Sports Med. 2008 May;36(5):949-55. Epub 2008 Apr 15.

8. Mithoefer K, Williams RJ 3rd, Warren RF, Potter HG, Spock CR, Jones EC, Wickiewicz TL, Marx RG. The microfracture technique for the treatment of articular cartilage lesions in the knee. A prospective cohort study.J Bone Joint Surg Am. 2005 Sep;87(9):1911-20

9. Peterson L, Brittberg M, Kiviranta I, Akerlund EL, Lindahl A. Autologous chondrocyte transplantation. Biomechanics and long-term durability.Am J Sports Med. 2002 Jan-Feb;30(1):2-12

10. Rodner CM, Adams DJ, Diaz-Doran V, Tate JP, Santangelo SA, Mazzocca AD, Arciero RA. Medial opening wedge tibial osteotomy and the sagittal plane: the effect of increasing tibial slope on tibiofemoral contact pressure. Am J Sports Med. 2006 Sep;34(9):1431-41. Epub 2006 Apr 24.

11. Ryan JA, Eisner EA, DuRaine G, You Z, Reddi AHJ. Mechanical compression of articular cartilage induces chondrocyte proliferation and inhibits proteoglycan synthesis by activation of the ERK pathway: implications for tissue engineering and regenerative medicine Tissue Eng Regen Med. 2009 Feb;3(2):107-16.

12. Spahn G, Kirschbaum S, Kahl E. Factors that influence high tibial osteotomy results in patients with medial gonarthritis: a score to predict the results. Osteoarthritis Cartilage. 2006 Feb;14(2):190-5.

13. Wang JH, Thampatty BP. Mechanobiology of adult and stem cells. Int Rev Cell Mol Biol. 2008;271:301-46.

"To study the phenomenon of disease without books is to sail on uncharted sea, while to study books without patients is not to go to the sea at all..."

(Sir William Osler)

Chapter 12.

Oats and Mega Oats. Why, When and How

Jochen Paul, Peter U. Brucker, Stephen Vogt, Andreas B. Imhoff

Take Home Message

The transplantation of articular cartilage with autologous and allogenic osteochondral grafts has shown promising results in the treatment of circumscribed osteochondral defects. Compared with bone-marrow stimulating techniques, osteochondral grafts provide repair with a hyaline articular cartilage matrix and viable chondrocytes potentially capable of maintaining the matrix. Several clinical studies indicate that these techniques can restore the articular surface of the joint. Only in limited cases a morbidity of the donor site is described.

Introduction

Autologous osteochondral transplantation (AOT) or OATS (Osteochondral Autograft Transfer System, Arthrex, Naples, FL, USA) is nowadays accepted as one of the major treatment options for cartilage defect repair. In particular in combination with subchondral bone damage, it is one of the favoured treatment options because the subchondral bone damage has to be repaired in combination with the cartilage to provide good results.

The OATS technique has been reported for multiple recipient sites including the knee, ankle, elbow, and shoulder joint. A combined hyaline cartilage and bone cylinder is harvested from a donor site (typically a non-weight bearing area of the knee joint) and transplanted into the defect area in an one-step surgical procedure. Usually, the main donor sites for OATS are the most proximal medial and lateral aspects of the femoral trochlea or the notch.

Patients with osteochondral lesions (OCL) typically present load-dependent pain of the affected joint. Conservative treatment is hardly successful in osteochondral lesions because the therapy is not causal and these lesions rarely heal spontaneously, especially in adults.

A stage adjusted evaluation of the osteochondral defect is essential for further therapeutic decision making. Imhoff et al.[7] developed a classification system for osteochondral lesions of the knee based on radiography, magnetic resonance imaging (MRI) and arthroscopic findings. Even if primarily designed for the knee joint, this classification system can be used for other joints as well.

The quality of the repair tissue is often discussed when different techniques for repair of osteochondral lesions are compared. Hyaline cartilage seems to provide the best biomechanical properties compared to other methods. Therefore it might preserve the joint from further damage or functional deterioration.

Contraindications:
• Osteoarthritis of the affected joint
• Chondrocalcinosis
• Uncorrectable ligamentous instabilities
• Malalignment of the mechanical axis
• Open growth plate
• Advanced age beyond the 5th decade or equivalent biological age

Imaging

Conventional radiographs in two (ankle, elbow) or three planes (knee, shoulder) are essential for adequate radiological diagnostics and verification of an OCL. However, radiologic imaging might be totally unremarkable because many OCLs are only detectable when there is a significant osseous defect. Therefore, if an OCL is clinically suspected, a MRI with intravenously applied contrast agent should be performed which represents the gold standard for diagnostics of an OCL.

A) Knee

Indication
Most frequently, osteochondral defects in the knee are found as idiopathic osteochondrosis dissecans at the medial femoral condyle. In adults, only symptomatic osteochondral defects should be treated with combined bone-cartilage transplantation. Accidentally diagnosed defects at the MRI may be monitored for

potential extension; however, an acute operative intervention is not required in most of these asymptomatic lesions.

Surgical technique

The OATS cylinders can be implanted in an open procedure or arthroscopically. Whenever possible, an arthroscopic procedure should be performed. The arthroscopic procedures are resulting in less morbidity, less infection rates, and smaller scars.

The patient should be also prepared for an alternative open procedure because some osteochondral defects may be inaccessible by arthroscopy. If the lesion is far posteriorly or if the knee cannot be extended or flexed sufficiently for adequate access, open surgery may be required. In the arthroscopic technique, portal selection and placement is crucial for perpendicular access with the "recipient chisel" to the lesion. Then, the osteochondral cylinder is harvested at the donor site from the proximolateral or proximomedial fermoral condyle. Using a guide sleeve, the harvested cylinder is placed into the defect in a press-fit technique. By arthroscopic visualization, the surface of the cylinder must be controlled to be well adapted to the surrounding cartilage without any protrusion.

Postoperative management

An individual postoperative regime according to the defect size and characteristics is applied. If the lesion is smaller than 2 cm^2 and the surrounding cartilage is stable, partial weight bearing (15 kg) can be implemented for the first 6 weeks. If the defect is larger and the skirt is unstable, non-weight bearing for 6 weeks should be performed. Passive motion of the knee joint starting from the first postoperative day is crucial for cartilage nutrition and can be applied by a continuous passive motion device (CPM). Conventional radiographs are taken on the first postoperative day in two planes; an MRI should only be performed in persistent symptomatic cases postoperatively

Results / actual literature

Chow et al.[5] evaluated 30 patients with a mean follow-up of 45 months after arthroscopic treatment of OCLs of the knee with autologous osteochondral transplantation. Postoperatively, the mean Lysholm score significantly improved from 43 points preoperatively to 87 points postoperatively. Good or excellent results were shown in 83% of the patients. In the IKDC assessment 87% of patients classified their knee as normal or nearly normal. Repeated arthroscopy with needle biopsy of the graft was performed in nine patients. Seven patients showed complete and two patients showed partial healing. The histological examination revealed viable chondrocytes and normal hyaline cartilage in the patients with complete healing. Congruency of the articular surface was restored in 92% of the patients.

B) Ankle

Indication
Approximately 85% of the OCLs are located on the medial aspect of the talus. However, medial OCLs are often associated with a lateral ankle sprain. The idiopathic osteochondrosis dissecans is a particular form of the OCL and is classified into five different stages[7]. Symptomatic osteochondral lesions at the ankle may be treated with an osteochondral transplantation to provide a sufficient osseous fundament for the cartilaginous layer. Concomitant subchondral cysts of the talus, which are often localized underneath the cartilage lesion can be addressed simultaneously with the OATS procedure.

Relative contraindication
Relative contraindications represent the age and the body mass index (BMI) of the patients. Because of inferior cartilage quality in patients with a biological age over 45, we are reluctant to perform OATS procedures in these patients. Obese patients present significantly more donor site morbidity at the knee joint as shown by Paul et al.[9].

Surgical technique
An anterolateral or anteromedial approach to the ankle is used dependent on the location of the lesion. If the OCL cannot be assessed by maximal plantar flexion, an additional osteotomy of the distal fibula or tibia is necessary. The defect has to be well exposed for exact measurement of the lesion size. Then the osteochondral lesion is excised with the "recipient chisel" (Figure 1). The "donor chisel" is used for graft harvesting from the proximolateral femur condyle using a separate anterolateral approach. The diameter of the "donor chisel" is slightly larger compared to the diameter of the "recipient chisel" (OATS, Arthrex, Naples FL, USA). The donor site cylinder is trimmed to an adequate height for press-fit fixation into the prepapred recipient socket. Special attention must be paid for a congruent surface of the cartilage part of the transplant to the adjacent cartilage (Figure 2). Cancellous bone grafting of the donor site defect at the knee joint is not necessary.

Postoperative management
In case of a malleolar or tibial osteotomy a splint is used for six weeks. Non-weight bearing of the leg is mandatory for the first six weeks postoperatively. After bone healing (6 weeks) the splint can be removed, free range of motion is allowed and progressive weight bearing of 10 kg/week is recommended for regaining full function of the ankle joint. Conventional radiographs of the ankle are taken on the first postoperative day in two planes. Similar to the OATS procedure in the knee joint, a routine MRI postoperatively is not necessary.

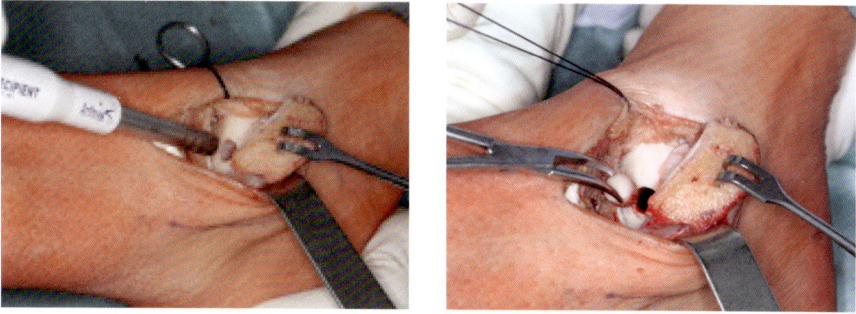

Figure 1: Left foot, medial approach and osteotomy of the medial malleolus. Harvesting of the osteochondral defect with the "recipient chisel" (OATS, Arthrex, Naples FL, USA). Figure 2: Insertion of the osteochondral plug, left foot, medial approach.

Results / actual literature

Actually, Kreuz et al.[8] described in more than 90% of transplanted osteochondral plugs good to excellent results following prior arthroscopic drilling. The AOFAS score increased significantly from 55 points preoperatively to 90 points postoperatively. Bone healing after tibial or fibular osteotomy and ingrowth of the transplant were without any complication in any case after 2 years follow-up. Baltzer et al.[2] also found in 43 patients good clinical results by increase of the Evanski and Waugh score from 52 to 88 points. Additionally, in a histological analysis of transplant biopsies intact hyaline cartilage was shown in all cases.

C) Elbow

Indication

Treatment of osteochondral lesions in the elbow remains challenging. Arthroscopic debridement, microfracturing, or retrograde drilling are often insufficient and provide only temporary relief with risk of subsequent osteoarthritis. Only an osteochondral transplantation procedure seems to provide the possibility to retain proper hyaline cartilage with an intact subchondral bone for repair of osteochondral lesions in the elbow (Figure 3). The joint congruity can be restored and the risk of osteoarthritis is possibly reduced.

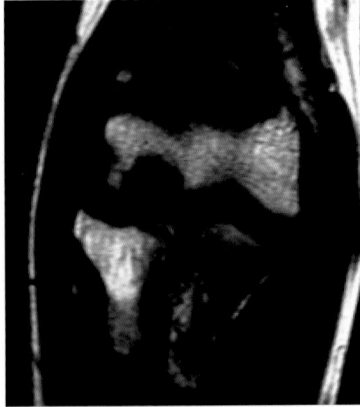

Figure 3: Preoperative MRI of right elbow revealing the isolated osteochondral defect of the capitellum.

Surgical technique

A dorsolateral approach with longitudinal incision from the radial epicondyle parallel to the olecranon and dorsal to the radial head is preferably choosen. The fascia is split between the anconeus muscle and M. extensor carpi ulnaris. The capsula is exposed and then opened dorsal to the radial head. For better exposition, the radial collateral ligament may have to be incised. Now the humero-radial joint is well exposed and by moving the joint in extension/flexion as well as rotation a thorough inspection is possible.

Usually, the defect in the capitellum is well exposed in full extension. The size of the lesion is measured and the defect is excised with a cylindrical bone plug using the aforementioned device (OATS, Arthrex, Naples, FL, USA). Subsequently, an osteochondral cylindrical donor graft is harvested from the non-weightbearing area of the proximolateral femoral condyle of the ipsilateral knee joint. The obtained cylinder of the chosen depth is then transplanted by press-fit technique into the recepient site of the elbow, carefully ensuring a good congruity of the chondral surface by proper placement (Figure 4).

If the donor cylinder is too long, it may be cut to the desired length, if it is too short, additional cancellous bone can be obtained from the donor site of the knee and fitted underneath the graft.

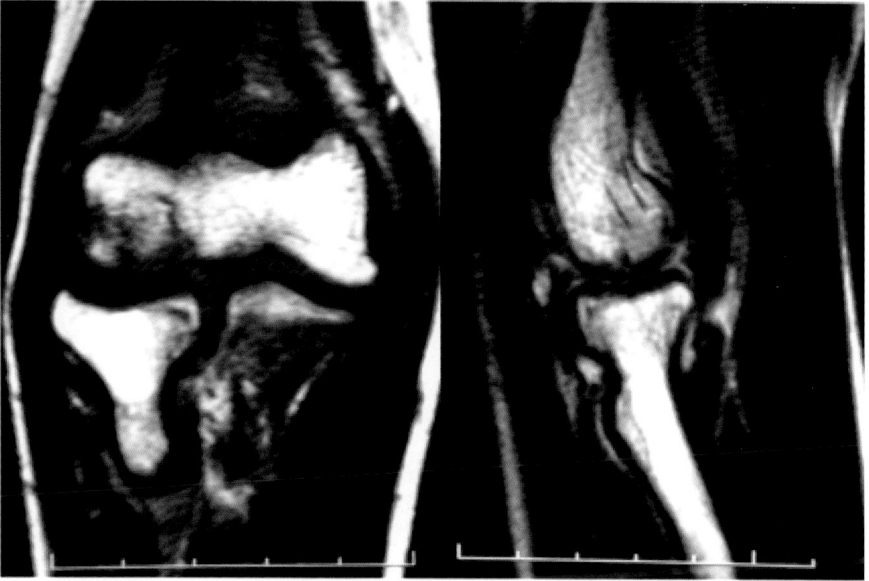

Figure 4: MRI of the capitellum 36 months postoperative demonstrates perfect ingrowth. Note the intact and congruent chondral surface of the graft.

Postoperative management

The postoperative regimen involves free range of motion, especially full flexion and extension for two weeks passively, followed by active free range of motion. Non-weight bearing or lifting of heavy loads for 6 weeks for the elbow and weight bearing for the knee as tolerated is allowed. Radiographs are taken on the first postoperative day, and MRI is optional 8-12 weeks after surgery (Figure 3).

Results / actual literature

Short- and midterm-results are encouraging[1]. The Broberg and Morrey score improved from a mean of 76 points preoperatively to 97 points postoperatively and pain scores were significantly reduced. Postoperative range of motion was free in all patients. No signs of osteoarthritis in any patient were seen in radiographs at the most recent follow-up. According to these results, the risk of a two joint procedure and the donor site morbidity seems justifiable.

Mega-OATS

Large osteochondral defects in the weight bearing zone of the medial or lateral femoral condyle especially in young patients are still a challenge for orthopaedic surgeons. Mosaicplasty represents a modification of the OATS technique by transplantation of multiple OATS plugs into the defect area[6]. However, this technique is limited due to the availability of the cylinders at the donor site. In addition, a restoration of the anatomic congruence of the cartilaginous surface and primary stability using multiple OATS plugs are technically demanding and often infeasible.

In the 1960's, the posterior femoral condyle of the knee was already recognized as a potential donor site for osteochondral tissue by Wagner[10]. The transfer of the posterior femoral condyle using an anterior approach was started in the 1990's at our department. The autologous Mega-OATS procedure represents a technical advancement of the posterior femoral condyle transfer. In contrast, the allogenic Mega-OATS technique illustrates an alternative procedure sparing the posterior femoral condyle as the donor site. Nevertheless in both autologous and allogenic Mega-OATS techniques, co-morbidities as malalignment and ligamentous instabilities must be addressed before or ideally simultaneously with the Mega-OATS intervention.

Indication

The indication criteria are similar to the OATS procedure; however, addressing the size of the osteochondral lesion is partially infeasible using a conventional single OATS technique or a press-fit technique due to a limited number of osteochondral plugs. Therefore, the Mega-OATS technique is an alternative procedure to the Mosaicplasty in which multiple osteochondral plugs are transplanted. Overall, the Mega-OATS technique must be appreciated as a salvage procedure for large osteochondral defects of the femoral condyles.

The indication criteria of the Mega-OATS procedure include:
• Large traumatic or posttraumatic osteochondral lesions
• Large osteochondral lesions with partial (grade III B according to Imhoff[7]) or complete detachment (grade IV B according to Imhoff[7]) and evidence of avital areas of the osteochondral fragment detected by intravenous Gadolinium enhanced MRI
• Focal osteonecrosis combined with limited cartilage defect size

Contraindication

The contraindication criteria for the Mega-OATS technique include:
• Osteoarthritis of the knee joint
• Chondrocalcinosis
• Uncorrectable ligamentous instabilities
• Uncorrectable deformity of the axis of the knee joint
• Open growth plate
• Advanced age beyond the 5th decade or equivalent biological age
• Profession or sports involving continuous or repetitive maximal loads with high knee flexion angles
• Limited compliance

Surgical Technique

In a supine position using a tourniquet, an anteromedial or anterolateral arthrotomy is performed due to the defect localization on the medial or lateral femoral condyle. The affected osteochondral area on the femoral condyle is exposed and measured (Figure 5).

According to the osteocartilaginous defect size and depth, the posterior femoral condyle is harvested by chisel osteotomy in a maximally flexed knee position. In detail, the direction of the posterior femoral condyle osteotomy is parallel or in elongation to the posterior cortex of the femoral diaphysis. Condyle or Hohmann retractors were used for protection of the neurovascular structures while performing the osteotomy. The Mega-OATS cylinder is harvested out of the removed posterior femoral condyle using a specially designed Mega-OATS workstation (Arthrex, Naples, FL, USA; Figure 6).

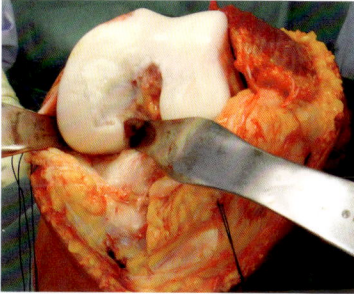

Figure 5: Left knee, anteromedial arthrotomy. Typical location of a large osteochondral defect in the weight bearing zone of the medial femoral condyle.

Usually, the diameter of the Mega-OATS cylinder is between 20 - 35 mm depending of the size of the osteochondral defect. A special recipient harvester and counter bore is utilized for reaming and preparation of the defect bed. The depth of the defect bed is dependent on the expansion of the osseous lesion detected by MRI. Intraoperatively, however, a correct drilling depth is accomplished by occurrence of bleeding subchondral surfaces within the defect socket. Finally, the Mega-OATS cylinder is placed into the recipient socket in a press-fit technique by consideration of an optimal congruence of the cartilaginous cylinder surface to the adjacent cartilage (Figure 7).

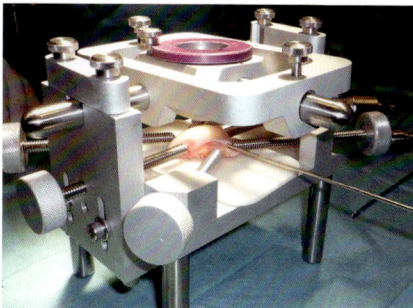

Figure 6: Specially designed workstation (Arthrex, Naples, FL, USA) for preparation of the Mega-OATS cylinder.

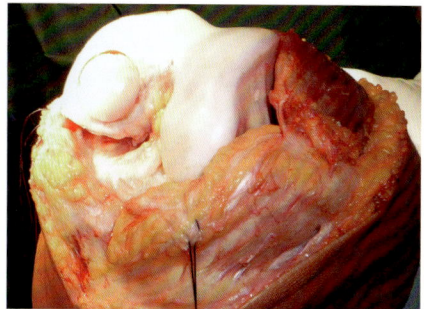

Figure 7: Intraoperative result following press-fit transplantation of the Mega-OATS cylinder into the prepared defect socket.

Postoperative Management

Postoperatively, unloading for 6 weeks using crutches is mandatory. Within this period, active range of motion is limited to flexion / extension 90°-0°-0° and supported by usage of a 4-point hard frame knee brace for at least 6 weeks. Continuous passive motion therapy and isometric muscle strengthening are concomitantly recommended. Beginning of the 7th week postoperatively, progressive loading with 20 kg per week and free active range of motion are allowed as tolerated until full weight bearing of the extremity is achieved. A progressive muscle and proprioceptive training starting after 3 months postoperatively for 12 weeks is performed. A specific sports rehabilitation program is started on the 7th month postoperatively (Brucker et al.[4]). Postoperative radiographs are undertaken following drain removal. MRI is optional, but not before 3 months postoperatively.

Results / actual literature

17 patients following transfer of the posterior femoral condyle according to the Mega-OATS procedure were clinically evaluated at an average follow-up of 12 months by Braun et al.[3]. In addition, 16 of 17 patients were re-evaluated at an average follow-up of 55 months including an image-guided evaluation protocol[3]. All patients had a large symptomatic osteochondral defect (average size 6 cm^2, range 4 - 9 cm^2) on the femoral condyle. In the Lysholm score, a significant increase of 62 points preoperatively to 85 points at 12 months and 81 points at 55 months postoperatively was found. At the primary follow-up of 12 months postoperatively, most of the patients complained about some discomfort of the operated knee in a static kneeling position and in a maximal squat position.

In 9 patients with varus malalignment, a simultaneous high tibial osteotomy was performed. However, a significant difference in the Lysholm score between the subgroup with and without simultaneous high tibial osteotomy could not be detected.

Overall, a highly subjective satisfaction rate could be found in more than 90 % of the patients. The postoperative level of recreational and amateur sports activities could be reached by 75% of the patients. In randomized MRI at the most recent follow-up, a good viability of the Mega-OATS graft as well as an intact posterior horn of the ipsilateral meniscus was observed.

References

1. Ansah, P., et al., Osteochondral transplantation to treat osteochondral lesions in the elbow. J Bone Joint Surg Am, 2007. 89(10): p. 2188-94.
2. Baltzer, A.W. and J.P. Arnold, Bone-cartilage transplantation from the ipsilateral knee for chondral lesions of the talus. Arthroscopy, 2005. 21(2): p. 159-66.
3. Braun, S., et al., The 5.5-year results of MegaOATS--autologous transfer of the posterior femoral condyle: a case-series study. Arthritis Res Ther, 2008. 10(3): p. R68.
4. Brucker, P.U., S. Braun, and A.B. Imhoff, [Mega-OATS technique--autologous osteochondral transplantation as a salvage procedure for large osteochondral defects of the femoral condyle]. Oper Orthop Traumatol, 2008. 20(3): p. 188-98.
5. Chow, J.C., et al., Arthroscopic autogenous osteochondral transplantation for treating knee cartilage defects: a 2- to 5-year follow-up study. Arthroscopy, 2004. 20(7): p. 681-90.
6. Hangody, L. and P. Fules, Autologous osteochondral mosaicplasty for the treatment of full-thickness defects of weight-bearing joints: ten years of experimental and clinical experience. J Bone Joint

Surg Am, 2003. 85-A Suppl 2: p. 25-32.

7. Imhoff, A.B. and U. König, Arthroscopic based staging of osteochondral lesions (OCL) of the knee. Diagnostic and classification. Arthroskopie, 2003. 16: p. 23-28.

8. Kreuz, P.C., et al., Mosaicplasty with autogenous talar autograft for osteochondral lesions of the talus after failed primary arthroscopic management: a prospective study with a 4-year follow-up. Am J Sports Med, 2006. 34(1): p. 55-63.

9. Paul, J., et al., Donor-site morbidity after autologous osteochondral transplant for lesions of the talus. J Bone Joint Surg Am, 2009. 91(7): p. 1683-1688.

10. Wagner, H., Operative Behandlung der Osteochondrosis dissecans des Kniegelenks. Z Orthop Grenzgeb, 1964. 98: p. 333-335.

*"The art of medicine consists in amusing
the patient while nature cures the disease"*

(Voltaire)

Chapter 13.

The Use of Platelet Rich Plasma for Cartilage Repair

Alberto Gobbi, Lorenzo Boldrini, Joao Espregueira-Mendes

Take Home Message

PRP represents a growing number of therapeutic applications with exciting and promising preliminary clinical results.
A standardization is warranted in terms of system of production, PRP characteristics, clinical indications, way of administration and therapeutic protocols until a more common use is recommended.

Introduction

The social impact of bone and cartilage pathologies entails high costs in terms of therapeutic treatments and loss of income. In the US osteoarthritis (OA) medicines cost $5.31 billion dollars in 2007, (Intercontinental Marketing Service data) and muscoloskeletal conditions including OA results in nearly $86.2 billion per year in direct medical expenses i.e. total joint replacement procedures and loss of income and production. Accordingly, 2000 to 2010 have been called the "decade of bone and joint" to launch global awareness and promote further research in prevention, diagnosis and treatment of joint injuries.
For these reasons, the trend of the research is now going towards preventive in-

terventions and therapeutic solutions that can lead to an enhancement of tissue regeneration and the reduction of degenerative mechanisms.

Cartilage Treatment

Hyaline cartilage is known for its specific characteristics that combine a smooth surface and the ability to withstand extreme amounts of pressures. It is extremely important to reconstruct a perfect surface that will withstand heavy loads; unfortunately articular cartilage lesions, with their inherent limited healing potential, remain a challenging problem for orthopaedic surgeons. In the last decade, the trend was to replace the articular surface with expensive and sophisticated implants when articular lesions become full blown OA but recent studies with the use of new ortho-biological techniques have been utilized in cartilage lesions with increasing frequency and effectiveness as a way to regenerate tissue homeostasis and retard progression of OA. Growth factors and mesenchymal stem cells have been used successfully in many medical fields such as maxillofacial, cosmetic, spine, orthopaedic and general wound healing applications.

Growth factors from platelet rich plasma (See Fig 1-3):

Recently the idea of "biological solution for biological problems" has lead to the development of less invasive procedures and accelerated treatments that in general reduce morbidity while enhancing functional recovery[1]. One interesting therapy is platelet-rich plasma (PRP) that can be defined as the volume of the plasma fraction from autologous blood with platelet concentration above baseline (200000 platelets/µl)[2]. Initially used as "platelet concentrate" in transfusion medicine to treat hemorrhagic conditions secondary to thrombocytopenia, acute leukaemia or severe blood loss after surgery, the use of blood derived products (fibrin glue) as wound sealant and stimulus for wound healing was started 40 years ago[3]. Ferrari et al. then first introduced it in 1987 in open-heart surgery to decrease bleeding[4]. Consequently Whitman described the use of platelet concentrate to replace fibrin glue and improve healing[5]. Later this therapy enjoyed a great increase in popularity because of the versatility, biocompatibility and low-costs of this approach and has stimulated its therapeutic use in many medical field. Scientific research and technology has provided new insight in understanding the biological potential of platelet in wound healing process[1,6,7].

It is well known that platelets have many functions beyond simple haemostasis; platelets contain many important bioactive proteins and growth factors, such as platelet-derived growth factor (PDGF), insulin-like growth factor (IGF-1), transforming growth factor (TGF-B), epidermal growth factor (EGF), fibroblast growth factor (bFGF), vascular endothelial growth factor (VEGF), and others. These factors when secreted, regulate key processes involved in tissue repair, including cell proliferation, chemotaxis, migration, cellular differentiation, and extracellular matrix synthesis[8,9]. The rationale for topical use of platelet-enriched preparations is to stimulate the natural healing cascade and tissue regeneration by a "supraphysiological" release of platelet-derived factors directly in the site of treatment. When PRP begin to work, the local tissue which is in contact with this preparation benefits from the particular actions of Growth Factors, able to interact with each other and individually with cell surface receptors and with different extracellular matrix proteins. Growth factors mediate the biological processes necessary for repair of soft tissues such as muscle, tendon and ligament following acute traumatic, or overuse injury, and animal studies have demonstrated clear benefits in terms of accelerated healing[10,11]. However which growth factors are more beneficial should be better understood. The complexity of interactions between different growth factors and the anabolic versus catabolic in vivo balance needs more evidence and scientific studies. Furthermore, Martinez et al.[12], in a recent search of electronical database, noted there are also little data about PRP safety. They also observed several methodological limitations and, consequently, future research should focus on strong and well-designed RCTs that assess the efficacy and safety of PRP.

There are various ways of delivering higher doses of growth factors to injured tissue, but each has in common, a reliance on release of growth factors from blood platelets. Platelets must be activated in order to release growth factors. For PRP-gel preparations platelets are normally activated by thrombin (autologous or from animals), Calcium Chloride and pro-coagulant enzyme i.e. Batroxobin (Plateltex®act, Regen Lab, Mollens VD)[13] which works as a fibrinogen cleaving enzyme inducing a rapid fibrin clot formation. PRP solutions injected directly for topic treatments are activated by local thrombin. In general, the amount of growth factors delivered is not necessarily proportional to the platelet count, because of the high variability of growth factors contained in platelet among individuals[14,15]. However studies have shown that clinical efficacy of PRP preparations can be expected at minimum 4 to 6 fold increase of platelets count from baseline value[16,17]. Final bio-availability growth factors is also dependent from extremely high sensitivity of platelets to process induced stress, from blood extraction to PRP gel preparation; furthermore the kinetic and release of growth factors from different PRP preparation can vary, even if it is still unclear if it can be clinically relevant[2].

PRP can be obtained from a simple blood extraction using the kit provided by the manufacturer. Once the blood is collected it will undergo a centrifugation process that will produce PRP.

Several systems are available to prepare the PRP and the platelet gel: however many differences exist between commercial PRP products. For scientific evaluation of platelet rich plasma efficacy in clinical studies a standardization of different PRP preparations is warranted. Dohan Ehrenfest et al.[18] proposed a classification in four categories, depending on leukocytes and fibrin content of PRP: leukocytes poor or pure platelet rich plasma (P-PRP), leukocytes and platelet rich plasma (L-PRP), leukocytes poor or pure platelet rich fibrin (P-PRF) and leukocytes and platelet rich fibrin (L-PRF). Products has been evaluated according to key parameters: preparation kits and centrifuge (size and weight of centrifuge, duration of procedure, cost and ergonomy), platelets and leucocyte (volume, collection efficiency and preservation and fibrin concentration (concentration, density and polymerization type). They concuded that the world of platelets concentrates for surgical use is actually a jungle of unclear products and we agree with them that a clarification is the first step in defining any clinical and biotechnological applications for each technique.

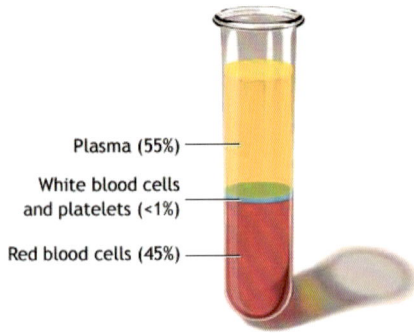

Figure 1: PRP

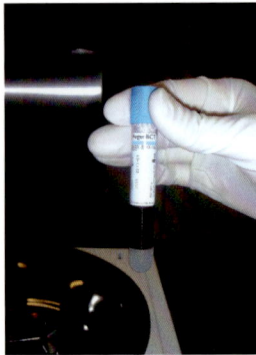

Figure 2: PRP preparation

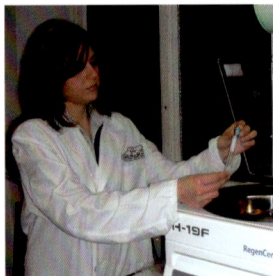

Figure 3: PRP preparation

Conservative Biological Approach to OA: PRP

Platelet rich plasma (PRP) preparations have been used both in surgical and out-patient procedures in the treatment of several muscoloskeletal problem with effective results[1,6]. Mishra et al.[19] suggested in their study that PRP treatment given to elbow epicondylar tendinosis patients prior to surgery can prevent the necessity to undergo the surgical procedure. Other studies reported clinical efficacy of PRP applications in soft tissue surgical and conservative treatments[19,21,22]. Furthermore, PRP combined with proper nutrition (control of BMI), exercise and lifestyle, can act as a preventive agent in chronic and degenerative muscoloskeletal disease[23].

Recent studies have documented the effectiveness of growth factors in chondrogenesis and preventing degeneration of the joints. Nakagawa et al.[24], has reported the in vitro efficacy of autologous PRP in stimulating the proliferation and collagen synthesis of human chondrocytes, suggesting the use of this method in the treatment of cartilage defects. Akeda et al.[25] successfully cultured porcine chondrocytes with PRP showing higher cell proliferation and proteoglycans and collagen synthesis. In animal studies Frisbie et al reported clinical and histologic improvement in osteoarthritis affected joints of horses after treatment with platelet rich plasma. Moreover Wu et al.[27] in an experimental study done on animals showed the effectiveness of intrarticular injections of PRP with chondrocytes grown in vivo that resulted in the formation of new cartilage tissue.

In clinical studies Anitua et al.[28] showed that an intra-articular injection of PRP could induce an increase in production of hyaluronic acid structure and promote angiogenesis and cell proliferation. Cugat et al.[29] used platelet-rich growth factors (PRGF) to treat chondral defect in athletes and obtained good results, according to their experiences for other connective tissue repair, they showed that PRGF in physiological concentration is effective for the recovery of connective tissue furthermore local treatment is safe and does not alter the systemic concentrations of these proteins. Kon et al.[30] have studied a group of 30 patients with symptomatic degenerative disease of the knee joints treated with three PRP intra-articular injections weekly; the follow up at 6 months showed positive effects on the function and symptoms with an improvement of 85% in scores evaluated for patients with median age less than 60 years, while in patients with age greater than 60 years, the improvement shown was only 30%. Same authors recently presented their comparative study between HA and PRP: 91 patients with a mean age of 50.1 years with degenerative lesions and OA were followed up after injection of HA or PRP. Results were better in PRP group in clinical knee scores and pain score[31].

In our institution we used a L-PRP according to Dohan Ehrenfest et al classification, in treating early arthritis. Among a group of 50 patients we treated with PRP injections we followed up 23 patients with a grade 3 and 4 chondral defects of the knee and a mean age of 44.3 years, 13 cases with previous knee surgeries. We collected pain visual analogue scale (VAS) and Knee Osteoarthritis Outcome Score (KOOS) at pre-treatment and 6-12 months post treatment; preliminary results are encouraging showing a trend towards improvement in both scores[32].

Finally several authors reported the use of growth factors and PRP preparations to stimulate mesenchymal stem cells (MSC) proliferation for chondrogenesis: Drengk et al.[33] reported in their in vitro study that platelet rich plasma has proliferative effects on autologous MSC and chondrocytes, suggesting advantages for one-step surgical procedure in cartilage transplantation using a combination of cells and growth factors. Mishra et al.[34] concluded in their study the PRP enhances MSC proliferation and suggest that PRP causes chondrogenic differentiation of MSC in vitro. These results were also evident in an in vivo study done by Milano et al.[35] that showed a more effective cartilage repair after microfracture associated to hydrogel scaffold with PRP. Nishimoto et al.[36] suggested that simultaneous concentration of PRP and bone marrow cells (BMC), acting as a sources of growth factors and "working cells", could play important roles in future regenerative medicine. This was supported by several authors[27,37,38] stating that growth factors could act like as a carrier to fix chondrocytes into cartilage defects and can be combined with mesenchymal stem cells. Buda et al.[39] reported the results of a group of patients treated with BMC and PRP at a same time in a collagen powder scaffold for grade 3 and 4 chondral lesion of the talus: at a mean follow up of 10 months AOFAS score improved compared to pre-op and 87.5% of patients were able to resume sport activity without complications.

Preliminary data are encouraging; however, further studies on clinical efficacy will clarify if simultaneous use of PRP and MSC could represent a real solution for regenerative medicine in cartilage repair.

Conclusions

Biological approaches to cartilage lesions is a new fascinating challenge; a number of viable options have been made available over the years to address problems concerning cartilage damage and each technique has its advantages and disadvantages.
PRP represents now a whole world of therapeutic applications with exciting and promising preliminary clinical results. However we believe that a standardization is warranted in terms of system of production, PRP characteristics, clinical indications, way of administration and therapeutic protocols. Moreover studies are currently under way to clarify some of the questions that still remain unanswered regarding the long-term durability of these procedures and the possible modifications that can still be done to achieve better results.
Biotechnology is progressing at a rapid pace, exploring new horizons and allowing the introduction of numerous products for clinical application. However, carefully conducted randomized prospective studies for each of these innovations should be carried out to validate the safety and efficacy in cartilage regeneration.

References

1. Anitua E, Sanchez M, orive G, Andia I. The potential impact of the preparation rich in growth factors (PRGF) in different medical fields. Biomaterials 2007;28:4551-4560
2. Mazzucco L, Balbo V, Cattana E, Guaschino R, Borzini P . Not every PRP-gel is born equal. Evaluation of growth factor availability for tissues through four PRP-gel preparations: Fibrinet®, RegenPRP-Kit®, Plateltex® and one manual procedure.Vox Sanguinis 2009 Apr 8. [in press]
3. Matras H. Die Wirkungen vershiedener Fibrinpreparate auf Kontinuitat-strennungen der Ratten-haut. Oster Z Stomatol 1970;6: 338-359
4. Ferrari M, Zia S,Valbonesi M. A new technique for hemodilution, preparation of autologous platelet-rich plasma and intraoperative blood salvage in cardiac surgery. Int J Artif Organs. 1987 ; 10 : 47-50.
5. Whitman, DH et al. Platelet gel: an autologous alternative to fibrin glue with application in oral and maxillofacial surgery. J Oral Maxillofac Surg 1997;55: 1294-1299
6. Sampson S, Gerhardt M, Mandelbaum B. Platelet rich plasma injection grafts for muscoloskeletal injuries: a review. Curr Rev Muscoloskelet Med 2008.
7. Nurden AT, Nurden P, Sanchez M, Andia I, Anitua E. Platelets and wound healing. Frontiers in Bio-science 2008; 13: 3525-3548
8. Bennett NT, Schultz GS. Growth factors and wound healing: biochemical properties of growth factors and their receptors. Am J Surg. 1993 Jun;165(6):728-37.
9. Molloy T, Wang Y, Murrell G. The roles of growth factors in tendon and ligament healing. Sports Med. 2003;33(5):381-94. Review.
10. Aspenberg P, Virchenko O. Platelet concentrate injections improves achilles tendon repair in rats. Acta Orthop Scand 2004;75(1): 93-99
11. Menetrey J, Kasemkijwattana C, Day CS, et al. Growth factors improves muscle healing in vivo. JBJS(Br) 2000; 82 (1): 131-137
12. Martínez-Zapata MJ, Martí-Carvajal A, Solà I, Bolibar I et al. Efficacy and safety of the use of au-tologous plasma rich in platelets for tissue regeneration: a systematic review. Transfusion. 2009 Jan;49(1):44-56.
13. Mazzucco L, Balbo V, Cattana E, Borzini P Platelet-rich plasma and platelet gel preparation using Plateltex. Vox Sang. 2008 Apr;94(3):202-8. Epub 2008 Jan 7
14. Borzini P. Mazzucco L. "Tissue regeneration and in-loco administration of platelet derivatives. Clinical outcome, heterogeneous products, heterogeneity of the effector mechanisms" Transfusion 2005; 35:1759-1767
15. Weibrich G, Kleis WKG, Hitzler WE, Hafner G. "Comparison of the platelet concentrate collection system with the plasma-rich-in-growth-factors kit to produce platelet-rich plasma: a technical re-port". Int J Oral Maxillofac Impants 2005; 20:118-123
16. Weibrich G, Hansen T, Kleis W, Buch R, Hitzler WE. Effect of platelet concentration in platelet rich plasma on peri-implant bone regeneration. Bone 2004; 34:665-671
17. Everts PA, Knape JT, Weibrich G, Schönberger JP, Hoffmann J, Overdevest EP, Box HA, van Zundert A. Platelet-rich plasma and platelet gel: a review. J Extra Corpor Technol. 2006 Jun;38(2):174-87. Re-view
18. Dohan Ehrenfest DM, Rasmusson L, Albrektssson T. Classification of platelet concentrates: from pure platelet-rich plasma (P-PRP) to leucocyte- and platelet-rich fibrin (L-PRF). Trends in Biothecnol-ogy, 2008; 27 (3): 158-167
19. Mishra A, Pavelko T.Treatment of chronic elbow tendinosis with buffered platelet-rich plasma. Am J Sports Med. 2006 Nov;34(11):1774-8. Epub 2006 May 30.
20. Randelli P, Arrigoni P, Cabitza P et al. Autologous platelet-rich plasma for arthroscopic rotator cuff repair. A pilot study. Disability and Rehabilitation 2008;30 (20-22): 1584-1589.
21. Kon E, Filardo G, Delcogliano M et al. Platelet-rich plasma: new clinical application. A pilot study for treatment of jumper's knee. Injury 2009; 40(6): 598-603
22. Anitua E, Sanchez M, Nurden AT et al. New insights into and novel applications for platelet rich and fibrin therapies. Trends in Biotechnology, 2006; 24(5):227-234
23. Gobbi A, Bathan L. Biological approaches for cartilage repair. J Knee Surg, 2009; 22(1): 36-44
24. Nakagawa K. Et al. Effects of autologous platelet-rich plasma on the metabolism of human articular chondrocytes. 7th World Congress of ICRS, Warsaw, October 2007
25. Akeda K, An HS, Okuma M. Platelet rich plasma stimulates porcine articular condrocyte prolifara-tion and matrix biosynthesis. Osteoarthritis Cartilage 2006; 14(12): 1272-1280
26. Frisbie D, Kawcak C, Werpy N, et al.. Clinical biochemical and histological effects of

intraarticular administration of autologous conditioned serum in horses with experimentally induced ostesoarthritis. Am J Vet Res 2007; 68(3):290-296.

27. Wu W, Chen F, Liu Y, Ma Q, Mao T. Autologous Injectable Tissue-Engineered Cartilage by Using Platelet-Rich Plasma: Experimental Study in a Rabbit Model. Journal of Oral and Maxillofacial Surgery, 2007 65 1951-1957

28. Anitua E. Et al. Platelet-released growth factors enhance the secretion of hyaluronic acid and leads hepatocyte growth factor production by synovial fibroblasts from arthritic patients. Rheumatology, 2007

29. Cugat R, Carrillo JM, Serra I, et al. Articular cartilage defects reconstruction by plasma rich growth factors. Basic science, clinical repair and reconstruction of articular cartilage defects: current status and prospects. TIMEO 801-807

30. Kon E. Utilisation of platelet-derived growth factors for the treatment of degenerative cartilage pathology. 7th World Congress of ICRS, Warsaw, October 2007

31. Kon E. Buda, Filardo G, et al. The Evolution of Arthritis: Growth Factors. Presented at XVII International Congress on Sports and Rehabilitation Traumatology. Bologna, Italy, April 2009

32. Boldrini, L. Gobbi, A. Infiltrative Treatment With Autologous Platelet Rich Plasma In Early Osteoarthritis: Our Experience. Presented at XVII International Congress on Sports and Rehabilitation Traumatology. Bologna, Italy, April 2009

33. Drengk A, Zapf A, Sturmer E, et al. Influence of Platelet – Rich Plasma on Chondrogenic Differentiation and Proliferation of Chondrocytes and Mesenchymal Stem Cells. Cells Tissues and Organs 2008 :10.1159.

34. Mishra A, Tummala P, King A et al. Buffered platelet-rich plasma enhances mesenchymal stem cell proliferation and chondrogenic differentiation. Tissue Eng Part C Methods. 2009 (in press).

35. Milano G, Zarelli D et al. Does Platelet Rich Plasma Injection enhance Cartilage Healing After Microfractures? An Animal Study. Poster no. 536. 54th Annual Meeting of the Orthopaedic Research Society.

36. Nishimoto S, Oyama T, Matsuda K.Simultaneous concentration of platelets and marrow cells a simple and useful technique to obtain source cells and growth factors for regenerative medicine. Wound Repair Regen. 2007 Jan-Feb;15(1):156-62

37. Espregueira-Mendes, J. Influence of Platelet Rich Plasma on Chondrogenic Differentiation and proliferation of chondrocytes.

38. Graziani F, Ivanovski S, Cei S, Ducci F, Tonetti M, Gabriele M. The in vitro effect of different PRP concentrations on osteoblasts and fibroblasts. Clin Oral Implants Res. 2006 Apr;17(2):212-9.

39. Buda R, Vannini F, Grigolo B et al. Tissue engeenering; surgical technique. G.I.O.T. 2007; 33 (Suppl).1) :S215-S222

"The success of a discovery depends upon the time of its appearance"

(S. Weir Mitchell)

Chapter 14.

Cartilage Defects-Osteochondral Allografts, Allogenic Chondrocytes and Allogenic Meniscal Transplants

Karl Fredrik Almqvist, Aad Dhollander, Peter Verdonk, René Verdonk

> ### Take Home Message
>
> *There is still a limited number of patients treated with allogenic chondrocytes and the short follow-up period the published results are so far only preliminary. However, the proposed approach with allogenic cells could be performed as a one-stage surgical procedure, in which an off-the-shelf product of phenotypically stable articular cartilage cells is used.*

Introduction

Autogenic repair techniques for cartilage defects include osteochondral plugs, microfracture and cartilage cell implantation. These techniques are the most widely accepted clinical treatment options for cartilage lesions due to the lack of immunogenic reactions. From 1987 on, autologous chondrocytes have been implanted in (osteo-)chondral lesions of the human knee[1]. In this technique cartilage is harvested from a non-weight-bearing area of the knee joint, e.g. the intercondylar notch or the edge of the trochlea, digested and the isolated chondrocytes are propagated in vitro in a monolayer culture condition. This procedure, proposed by Brittberg et al. in 1994 and called autologous chondrocyte implantation (ACI), is gaining wide scientific and clinical support for use in the repair of focal articular cartilage defects[1]. ACI presents some theoretical advantages over other cartilage reconstructive techniques such as autologous or allograft osteochondral transplantation, e.g. the reduced donor site morbidity and no treatment limitations related to defect size[2]. However, a number of problems can be observed with the standard first and second-generation ACI techniques. These include the difficulty in handling a delicate liquid suspension of chondrocytes at implantation surgery, the need to construct a watertight periosteum or collagen synthetic membrane seal using sutures, the need of a second open operative procedure, and possible complications such as hypertrophy related to the use of a periosteal flap[3]. More importantly, during in vitro propagation of the chondrocytes, dedifferentiation of the cells can occur and afterwards, these fibroblast-like chondrocytes show different biosynthetic properties than the original cartilage cells in the knee joint[4]. The use of large numbers of instantaneously delivered allogenic cartilage cells, mesenchymal autologous progenitor cells or osteochondral allografts could solve these last two problems[5].

Osteochondral autografts or mosaicplasty is an accepted technique for smaller defects, but its use is limited by the amount of available nonarticulating or non-weight-bearing cartilage and the possible presence of donor site morbidity[4-6]. Here as well, the use of allogenic osteochondral allografts could provide an advantage when large cartilage defects are to be treated.

Cartilage defects are often associated with a meniscal lesion. A (sub-)total meniscectomy may result in a painful knee with subsequent progressive osteoarthritis. These patients, often of a young age, could be helped with a meniscal allograft transplantation.

Allogenic Chondrocytes

Due to the many practical limitations associated with autologous tissue, the use of allogenic tissue has been considered as a possible alternative to successfully generate cartilage tissue. The avascularity of articular cartilage has led to the belief that the tissue is "immunoprivileged", although it has been reported that chondrocytes and their extracellular matrix (ECM) contain antigens (eg. type II, IX and XI collagen, and proteoglycans) that can be immunogenic[6,7]. There is evidence demonstrating that allogenic transplantation of isolated chondrocytes elicits an immune response, gradually destroying the resulting cartilage tissue[8,9]. In use of these relatively poor results of isolated allogenic chondrocytes transplantation and the more promising outcome of osteochondral allografting in vivo, transplantation of allogenic cartilage cells with natural or synthetic scaffolds has been investigated as an alternative for the repair of cartilage lesions. In animal models natural scaffolds, such as collagen and agarose, have been successfully used for allogenic transplantation without any signs of immunological reactions. Their compressive stiffness and histology is similar to native cartilage tissue for up to 19 months[10-12].

Previous research showed that human chondrocytes keep their phenotype in alginate with neosynthesis of an extracellular cartilage matrix and that this chondrocyte/alginate culture set-up can be biologically frozen without any impairment overall aggrecan synthesis rates or its cartilage-specific aggrecan subtypes once thawed[13]. In order to construct a ready-for-use implant for the treatment of focal cartilage lesions, primary human articular chondrocytes were cultured in vitro in alginate beads surrounded by fibrin gel for a period of eight weeks[14]. Because optimal cell proliferation rates and synthesis of ECM substances by the implanted chondrocytes in the temporary scaffold are essential, optimal concentrations of alginate and fibrin gel were searched for. The outgrowth of the cells from the alginate beads into the surrounding, initially cell-free fibrin gel was regularly investigated with immunohistochemistry for aggrecan, and type I and II collagen, both in the alginate and in the surrounding fibrin gel. This pilot study showed a strong presence of cells staining for aggrecan and type II collagen in 1% alginate from 1 week up to 8 weeks, and a progressive increase of outgrowing cells staining positive for aggrecan and type II collagen in the surrounding fibrin gel[14].

In the present study a biodegradable, alginate-based biocompatible scaffold containing human allogenic chondrocytes was used for the treatment of chondral and osteochondral lesions in the knee (Fig. 1-3)[15].

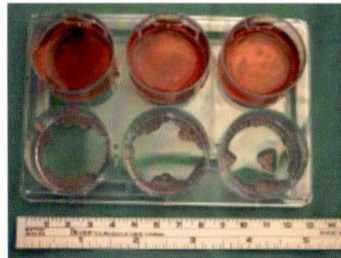

Figure 1: Alginate beads containing human allogenic chondrocytes, before (top) and after (bottom) removal of the nutrient medium.

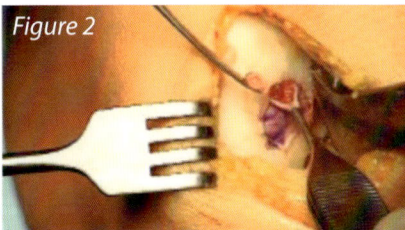

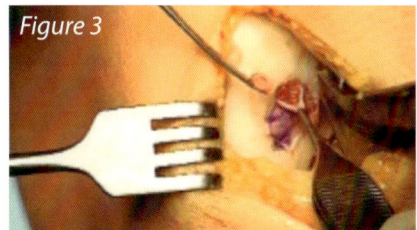

Figure 2: The alginate beads are inserted manually under the periosteal (or collagen i/III) flap. Figure 3: Sutured periosteal flap sealing the alginate beads in the cartilage defect.

The implantation of alginate beads containing human allogenic chondrocytes has been developed and performed at our department from 2002 on. We report the first clinical and histological results obtained in 21 patients after 24 months of follow-up.

The patients who participated in this study showed a strong gradual clinical improvement after surgery, as appeared from the significantly improved WOMAC and VAS pain scores 3 months after allogenic chondrocyte implantion. The rate of improvement was slightly slower for the WOMAC stiffness and physical function scores, which significantly improved after 6 months and, together with the other clinical variables, continued to improve during the 24 months of follow-up.

24 months after implantation of the alginate beads containing human allogenic chondrocytes, the WOMAC scores decreased by 86.5% in the present study. Compared with the results achieved by Knutsen et al.[16] and by Minas[17], our results suggest that the patients who participated in this study experienced more clinical symptoms before surgery and less 2 years after the procedure.

Osteochondral Allografts

As for the use of allogenic chondrocytes, the risk of transmittable diseases has to be taken into account when using (fresh) osteochondral allografts. Meticulous screening for bacteria and for HIV, hepatitis B/C, and other transmittable diseases by DNA polymerase chain reaction has to be performed before the osteochondral graft is released for clinical use.

Performing osteochondral allografting in the treatment of (large) cartilage defects permits the implantation of a graft with the appropriate size, contour and thickness of cartilage when it is obtained from an appropriately selected organ donor and area of the donor joint (Fig. 4). Initially frozen osteochondral allografts were used for reconstruction in orthopaedic tumor surgery[18], which prolonged the storage period and decreased the immunogenicity but also decreased the chondrocyte viability.

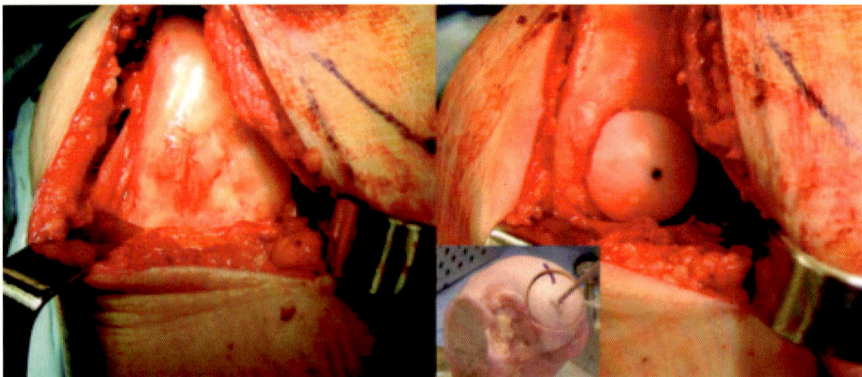

Figure 4: An example of a fresh osteochondral allograft (right) implanted into a major osteochondral defect (left) after debridement of the lesion. Insert: preparation of the osteochondral allograft from the same site as the defect in the patient.

To avoid the chondrocyte cell death in these osteochondral grafts, fresh osteo-chondral grafts are nowadays used and implantated within some weeks after harvesting. Good long-term clinical results have been reported using this tech-nique in the treatment of cartilage defects[19,20]. With a stable osseous graft base, the hyaline cartilage portion of the allograft can survive and function for 25 years or more[21].

Meniscal Allografts

Cartilage defects are often associated with meniscal tears. If the involved knee joint has a meniscal deficiency, a restoration of the meniscus should be per-formed before any cartilage defect is treated. The meniscus plays an important role in the complex biomechanics of the knee joint. It has functions in load bear-ing, load transmission, shock absorption, joint stability, joint lubrication, and joint congruity. Removal of this important anatomical structure eventually leads to degenerative changes of the articular cartilage[22-24]. Therefore, meniscal tissue should be preserved whenever possible. When the meniscus has been complete-ly lost, transplantation of a meniscal allograft has been a therapeutic option with favorable results, in terms of pain reduction and functional improvement, in the medium and long-term results[25-28]. These improvements are presumably due to an increase in contact area and thus a decrease in contact peak stresses ompared with these in a meniscectomized knee[29-32]. While decreases in contact stresses can result in pain relief and improved function, there is no reasonable proof that delayed meniscal transplantation prevents or slows cartilage degeneration in either compartment[27,33]. Few medium-term or long-term reports on meniscal al-lograft transplantations are available. In our department a survival analysis was carried out at a minimum of two years after our first 100 procedures involving transplantation of a viable meniscal medial or lateral allograft (Fig. 5)[34].
In this study, we presented the results of a survival analysis of the clinical out-comes of our first 100 procedures involving transplantation of viable medial and lateral meniscal allografts performed in ninety-six patients. Thirty-nine medial and sixty-one lateral meniscal allografts were evaluated after a mean of 7.2 years. Survival analysis was based on specific clinical end points, with failure of the al-lograft defined as moderate occasional or persistent pain or as poor function. An additional survival analysis was performed to assess the results of the sixtynine procedures that involved isolated use of a viable allograft (twenty of the thirty-nine medial allograft procedures and forty-nine of the sixty-one lateral allograft procedures) and of the thirteen viable medial meniscal allografts that were im-planted in combination with a high tibial osteotomy in patients with initial varus malalignment of the lower limb. Overall, eleven (28%) of the thirty-nine medial allografts and ten (16%) of the sixty-one lateral allografts failed. The mean cumu-lative survival time (11.6 years) was identical for the medial and lateral allografts. The cumulative survival rates for the medial and lateral allografts at ten years were 74.2% and 69.8%, respectively. The mean cumulative survival time and the cumulative survival rate for the medial allografts used in combination with a high tibial osteotomy were 13.0 years and 83.3% at ten years, respectively.

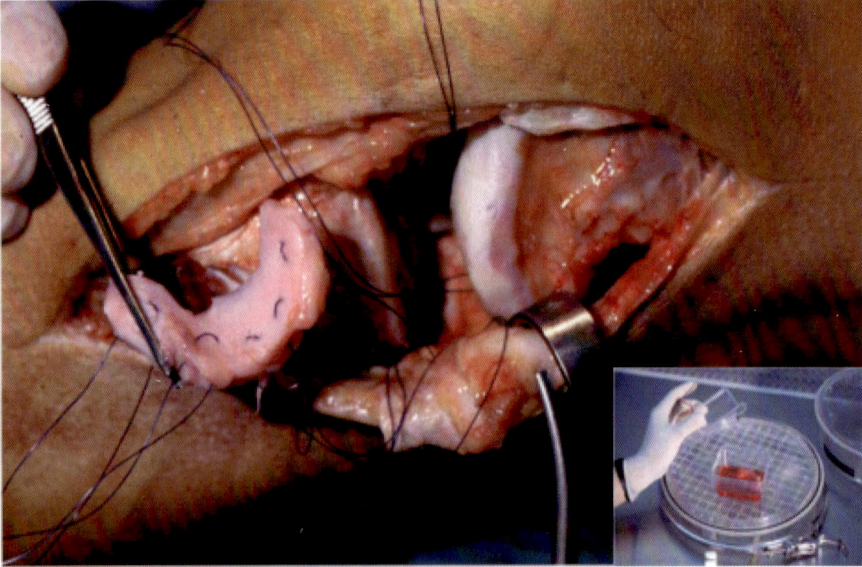

Figure 5: A meniscal allograft implanted after arthrotomy of the knee joint and sutured to the remnant of the meniscal rim. Insert: meniscal allograft transplant cultured in nutrient medium in the laboratory.

Conclusions: Transplantation of a meniscal allograft can significantly relieve pain and improve function of the knee joint. Survival analysis showed that this beneficial effect remained in approximately 70% of the patients at ten years.

Conclusion

The surgical procedure using allogenic chondrocytes in a scaffold or osteochondral allografts for the treatment of cartilage defects in humans shows promising clinical and histological results, based on our own experience and on the literature on osteochondral allografts. Both approaches involve a one-stage surgical procedure, in which an off-the-shelf product (allogenic chondrocytes in the matrix or osteochondral allograft) of phenotypically stable articular cartilage cells is used. Because of the limited number of patients treated with allogenic chondrocytes and the short follow-up period the presented results are only preliminary. The proposed approach could be performed as a one-stage surgical procedure, in which an off-the-shelf product of phenotypically stable articular cartilage cells is used. This allogenic cartilage cell procedure should ultimately resolve our failure to consistently reproduce hyaline cartilage repair tissue. Viable meniscal allograft transplantation can significantly relieve pain and improve function of the knee joint in the patient with a painful meniscectomized knee joint. Long-term and randomized controlled studies are mandatory to confirm the initial results and the reliability of the allogenic chondrocyte and the viable meniscal allograft transplantation procedure.

References

1. Brittberg M., Lindahl A., Nilsson A., Ohlsson C., Isaksson O., Peterson L. Treatment Of Deep Cartilage Defects In The Knee With Autologous Chondrocyte Transplantation. N Engl J Med, 1994, 331, 889-95.
2. Peterson L, Brittberg M., Kiviranta I., Åkerlund E.L., Lindahl A. Autologous chondrocyte transplantation. Biomechanics and long-term durability. Am J Sports Med, 2002, 30, 2-12.
3. Sgaglione N., Miniaci A., Gillogly S., Carter T.R. Update on advanced surgical techniques in the treatment of traumatic focal articular cartilage lesions in the knee. Arthroscopy, 2002, 18, 9-32.
4. Benya P.D., Schaffer J.D. Dedifferentiated chondrocytes reexpress the differentiated collagen phenotype when cultured in agarose gels. Cell, 1982, 30, 215-24.
5. Almqvist K.F. Human differentiated articular cartilage cells in biodegradable matrices. Preparative studies for their use in the repair of cartilage defects. A thesis submitted for fulfilment of the requirements for the degree: 'Doctor in the Medical Sciences'. Ghent, Belgium, 2001.
6. Bolano L., Kopta J.A. The immunology of bone and cartilage transplantation. Orthopedics, 1991, 14, 987-96.
7. Moskalewski S., Hyc A., Osiecka-Iwan A. Immune response by host after allogenic chondro-cyte transplant to the cartilage. Microsc Res Tech, 2002, 58, 3-13.
8. Malejczyk J., Osiecka A., hyc A., Moskalewski S. Effect of immunosuppression on rejection of cartilage formed by transplanted allogenic rib chondrocytes in mice. Clin Orthop Relat Res, 1991, 269, 266-73.
9. Malejczyk J., Moskalewski S. Effect of immunosuppression on survival and growth of cartilage produced by transplanted allogenic epiphyseal chondrocytes. Clin Orthop Relat Res, 1988, 232, 292-303.
10. Wakitani S., Nawata M., Tensho K., Okabe T., Machida H., Ohgushi H. Repair of articular carti-lage defects in the patello-femoral joint with autologous bone marrow mesenchymal cell transplantation: three case reports involving nine defects in five knees. J Tissue Eng Regen Med, 2007, 1, 74-9.
11. Masuoka K., Asazuma T., Ishihara M., Sato M., Hattori H., Yoshihara Y., Matsui T., Takase B., Kikuchi M., Nemoto K. Tissue engineering of articular cartilage using an allograft of cultured chondrocytes in a membrane-sealed atelocollagen honeycomb-shaped scaffold ACHMS scaffold). J Biomed Mater Res B Appl Biomater, 2005, 75, 177-84.
12. Rahfoth B., Weisser J., Sternkopf F., Aigner T., Vonder Mark K., Brauer R. Transplantation of allograft chondrocytes embedded in agarose gel into cartilage defects of rabbits. Osteoarthritis Cartilage, 1998, 6, 50-65.
13. Almqvist K.F., Wang L., Broddelez C., Veys E.M., Verbruggen G. Biological freezing of human articular chondrocytes. Osteoarthritis Cartilage, 2001, 9, 341-50.
14. Almqvist K.F., Wang L., Wang J., Baeten D., Cornelissen M., Verdonk R., Veys E.M., Verbruggen G. Culture of chondrocytes in alginate surrounded by fibrin gel: characteristics of the cells over a period of eight weeks. Ann Rheum Dis, 2001, 60, 781-90.
15. Almqvist K.F., Dhollander A., Verdonk P., Verdonk R., Verstraete K., Huysse W., Verbruggen G. The treatment of cartilage defects in the knee using alginate beads containing human allo-genic chondrocytes : preliminary results. Am J Sports Med, 2009, 37, 1920-9.
16. Knutsen G., Engebretsen L., Ludvigsen T.C., Drogset J.O., Grondtvedt T., Solheim E., Strand T., Roberts S., Isaksen V., Johansen O. Autologous chondrocyte implantation compared with microfracture in the knee. A randomized trial. J Bone Joint Surg Am, 2004, 86, 455-64.
17. Minas T. Autologous chondrocyten implantation for focal chondral defects of the knee. Clin Orthop Relat Res, 2001, 391, 349-61.
18. Tomford W.W., Springfield D.S., Mankin H.J. Fresh and frozen articular cartilage allografts. Orthopedics, 1992, 15, 1183-8.
19. Mcculloch P.C., Kang R.W., Sobhy M.H., Hayden J.K., Cole B.J. Prospective evaluation of pro-longed fresh osteochondral allograft transplantation of the femoral condyle: minimum 2-year follow-up. Am J Sports Med, 2007, 35, 411-20.
20. Görtz S., Bugbee W.D. Allografts in articular cartilage repair. J Bone Joint SurgAm, 2007, 88, 1374-84.
21. Grossa.E., Kim W., Las Heras F., Backstein D., Safir O., Pritzker K.P.H. Fresh osteochondral allografts for posttraumatic knee defects. Long-term followup. Clin Orthop Relat Res, 2008, 466, 1863-70.
22. Fairbank T.J. Knee joint changes after meniscectomy. J Bone Joint Surg Br, 1948, 30, 664-70.
23. Chatain F., Adeleine P., Chambat P., Neyret P.; Societe Francaise d'Arthroscopie. A comparative study of medial versus lateral arthroscopic partial meniscectomy on stable knees: 10-year minimum follow-up. Arthroscopy, 2003, 19, 842-9.

24. Englund M., Roos E.M., Lohmander L.S. Impact of type of meniscal tear on radiographic and symptomatic knee osteoarthritis: a sixteen-year followup of meniscectomy with matched controls. Arthritis Rheum, 2003, 48, 2178-87.

25. Wirth C.J., Peters G., Milachowski K.A., Weismeier K.G., Kohn D. Long-term results of meniscal allograft transplantation. Am J Sports Med, 2002, 30, 174-81.

26. Van Arkel E.R., De Boer H.H. Human meniscal transplantation. Preliminary results at 2 to 5-year follow-up. J Bone Joint Surg Br, 1995, 77, 589-95.

27. Dehaven K.E. Meniscus repair. Am J Sports Med, 1999, 27, 242-50.

28. Rath E., Richmond J.C., Yassir W., Albright J.D., Gundogan F. Meniscal allograft transplanta-tion. Two- to eight-year results. Am J Sports Med, 2001, 29, 410-4.

29. Paletta G.A. Jr, Manning T., Snell E., Parker R., Bergfeld J. The effect of allograft meniscal replacement on intra-articular contact area and pressures in the human knee. A biomechanical study. Am J Sports Med, 1997, 25, 692-8.

30. Huang A., Hull M.L., Howell S.M.. The level of compressive load affects conclusions from sta-tistical analyses to determine whether a lateral meniscal autograft restores tibial contact pressure to normal: a study in human cadaveric knees. J Orthop Res, 2003, 21, 459-64.

31. Chen M.I., Branch T.P., Hutton W.C. Is it important to secure the horns during lateral meniscal transplantation? A cadaveric study. Arthroscopy, 1996, 12, 174-81.

32. Alhalki M.M., Howell S.M., Hull M.L. How three methods for fixing a medial meniscal autograft affect tibial contact mechanics. Am J Sports Med, 1999, 27, 320-8

33. Aagaard H., Jorgensen U., Bojsen-Moller F. Immediate versus delayed meniscal allograft transplantation in sheep. Clin Orthop, 2003, 406, 218-27.

34. Verdonk P.C.M., Demurie A., Almqvist K.F., Veys E.M., Verbruggen G., Verdonk R. Transplan-tation of viable meniscal allografts. Survivorship and clinical outcome of one hundred cases. J Bone Joint Surg Am, 2005, 87, 715-24.

"Eyes, ears, nose and palpating fingers are the gem of physician, intact brain is the necklace!"

(Hippocrates)

Chapter 15.

Microfracture and Autologous Chondrocyte Implantation: Their Place in Therapy

Gunnar Knutsen

Take Home Message

Both microfracture and ACI have documented satisfactory clinical outcome. Lack of randomised studies including non operative control groups is a major weakness.
Today microfracture as a low cost and low morbidity procedure should be the preferred first line treatment for contained defects located on the medial/lateral femoral condyle and tibia.
For defects larger than 4 cm² ACI or other procedures involving periosteum, membranes or scaffolds may be a better option.

Introduction

Over the last two decades we have seen an enormous increase in the interest in biological repair of full-thickness articular cartilage defects. Cartilage defects are common; however, the impact and long term consequence for the affected joint are not well enough studied. Over time cartilage defects may lead to earlier onset of osteoarthritis. Thirty-forty years ago the main repair techniques were based on open debridement and drilling procedures, and this period was also the start of the successful era using artificial joint prosthesis for more advanced joint damage. However, joint replacement is not a good option for younger active patients with cartilage problems and surgeons worldwide are performing different types of cartilage surgery in order to improve symptoms and hopefully delay the development of disabling osteoarthritis needing an artificial joint.

Autologous chondrocyte implantation introduced the orthopaedic community to tissue engineering principles in clinical use, and the NEJM paper had a huge positive impact on the development in this field and it also created debate[1]. In the same period the microfracture technique gained popularity as a low-cost one stage procedure resulting in acceptable clinical results that were better than previous drilling procedures[2]. Microfracture and ACI are both in principle cell based therapies in contrast to osteochondral transfer techniques. The latter is moving cylinder(s) of healthy cartilage and bone from one location to the defect. The technique has limitations because of donor problems and lack of integration.

I have been using both techniques, ACI and Microfracture, since the mid nineties. I am also the project leader of the Norwegian randomised controlled study comparing ACI and microfracture[3,4]. My opinion is that as an orthopaedic surgeon you presently have good opportunities for attempting biological repair of cartilage defects if you have both ACI and microfracture options available for your patients. This includes newer generations of both techniques. Having no intention to present a new review regarding these methods, I will comment on aspects of the techniques and point to main results from our own study[3,4] and recent reviews found in the literature[5-9], and based on that I will give my recommendations for the use of microfracture and ACI in therapy.

Surgeons like Haggart and Magnussen in the forties and Pridie in the fifties used open debridement, abrasio and drilling for cartilage repair. The drilling procedure was popularised by Kenneth Hampden Pridie (1906-1963) and years after the technique got the name Pridie drilling. The results reported by Pridie have to be compared to what we achieve today. He quoted that 77% of his patients were satisfied with their operation and 64% were rated as good at follow up after mean 6.5 years[10.]

More than 20 years ago Steadman introduced arthroscopic microfracture as a modern modification of previous marrow stimulation procedures[2]. It consists of accurate debridement of the defect including the calcified layer. Unstable or delaminated cartilage has to be removed including the calcified layer and it is important to have a stable perpendicular edge around the defect. This accurate debridement has to be stressed because operations are still performed with too little aggressive cleaning, thus resulting in bad outcomes despite opening up for marrow elements by using designed microfracture tools or less favourable drills or pins. Shavers, spoons and curettes are important tools in preparing the defect. To be able to cut the anterior part of the defect a thin osteotome or anterior-posterior spoon is useful. An arthroscopic awl is then used to make multiple holes starting around the periphery and finishing in the middle of the defect. The picks should be 3-4 mm apart avoiding that they break into another. Marrow elements including bone marrow stem cells and growth factors will probably be important contributors in the clot filling the defect. Normally it is not necessary to use compression for bloodless surgery; local anaesthesia containing adrenaline in combination with the fluid pump will control the bleeding. It is important not to flush out the so called "super clot" and therefore other procedures should be performed before microfracture is finishing the operation (Fig 1).

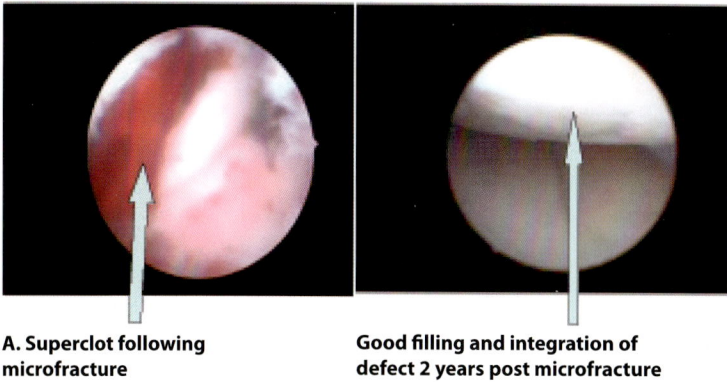

A. Superclot following microfracture

Good filling and integration of defect 2 years post microfracture

Figure 1: Microfracture.

Steadman also pointed to the importance of rehabilitation following this operative therapy. Localisation and size of defect are influencing the rehabilitation protocol. Microfracture has low morbidity and it is important that the patients are not overloading the treated knee over the first eight weeks. The weakest point, in my opinion, following microfracture is the relative instability of the clot. This has lead to newer generations of microfracture procedures where the clot is protected by periosteum, a covering membrane or a scaffold soaking up the cells from the subchondral bone. Steadman reported that at seven years after classic microfracture procedure, 80% of the patients rated them selves as improved[2]. Critics have been that the repair tissue is mainly fibrocartilage and results will diminish over time.

Autologous chondrocyte implantation started a new era in orthopaedics. May be some of us were too enthusiastic in the beginning and hoped that this was the ultimate solution for cartilage repair. Today we have realised that there is a long way to follow before we are able to reproducible regenerate functional and normal hyaline cartilage in adults. Nevertheless the era started by ACI was an important step forward. Tissue engineering has been established in orthopaedic surgery and the developments in this direction will not stop. Hyaline cartilage, lacking blood vessels, nerves and lymphatic drainage is a very specialized tissue containing few cells. It is possible that the regeneration of hyaline cartilage in humans is more difficult than the regeneration of other connective tissues.

ACI has been performed worldwide approximately more than 30000 times and has been established as a relative common procedure for repairing cartilage defects. Traditional ACI is a two step procedure. The first arthroscopic procedure includes biopsies (ca. 200mg) of healthy cartilage from a non-weight bearing area. The biopsies are prepared in the laboratory so that the chondrocytes are isolated and expanded in cell cultures. The second operation involves traditional open surgery. Accurate debridement and stabilisation of the cartilage edges are important part of this procedure like in other cartilage repairing procedures. Periosteum is harvested (from proximal tibia or distal femur) and sutured to the defect with fine resolvable sutures. Final sealing is achieved using fibrin-glue. It is important to create a watertight chamber underneath the periosteum where the expanded cells are injected. Most rehabilitation protocols use continued passive motion postoperatively and partial weight bearing for the first eight weeks.

Evidence based medicine has gained popularity in orthopaedic surgery. Historically surgeons have done what they have learned from senior colleagues, plus what they have learned from their own experience and mistakes. Randomised controlled trials (RCT) having enough power are difficult to perform in surgery, however; to move forward we need RCT and long term follow up as an important supplement to registers and retrospective studies. A Cochrane review[11] did not find evidence for superiority of any of the studied techniques for cartilage repair. Another paper by Jakobsen et al.[7] concluded that the majority of studies on cartilage had a low methodological quality. Recently a systematic review of the treatment of focal articular cartilage defects in the knee was published[8]. Authors of this paper identified five RCT and concluded that no technique consistently had superior results compared with the others. A weakness of all studies was that no control (nonoperative) groups were used. Our Norwegian study[3,4] had the highest Coleman score (least Bias) among these studies. Not included in the above mentioned review paper by Magnussen et al is the recently published RCT study comparing characterized chondrocyte (expanded population of chondrocytes, that expresses a gene score predictive to form hyaline-like cartilage in vivo) implantation and microfracture[12]. This multicenter study included biopsies from repair sites at one year using computerized histomorphometry and blinded overall histological evaluation. Clinical outcome scores were reported preoperatively and at 12 and 18 months following surgery. This well organised and performed study demonstrated that the repair tissue following Characterised Chondrocyte Implantation (CCI) was superior to that after microfracture, however, clinical outcomes were similar. These findings can be compared to the results from our randomised study having similar clinical outcomes for both treatment groups. However, this study included relatively small defects (2.5 cm^2) compared to our study (4.8 cm^2). In our study we also included more chronic cases.

At five years we had nine failures in each group (23%). Most of the failures occurred between two and five years after surgery. In our study we demonstrated a tendency (p= 0.008) for ACI to result in a more hyaline repair cartilage than the microfracture procedure, but this was not a significant finding with the numbers available. At five years we found that none of the patients having a failure had the best quality cartilage. This finding suggests that a predominant hyaline repair at two year may reduce the risk of later failure. However, we were unable to find any association between the histological quality of the repair tissue and clinical outcome. Overall 72% of our patients had less pain and 80% had a better Lysholm scores compared with baseline. Younger and more active patients had better clinical outcome scores.

What conclusions and recommendations can be given regarding ACI and microfracture in therapy? In general we still have to be cautious regarding strict flowcharts for surgical treatments for full-thickness cartilage defects. Surgical training/experience and available options are important factors in choosing the best treatment for our patients. Only symptomatic defects should have extensive surgery. Smaller defects discovered at arthroscopy can be minor debrided in the first setting. Non operative treatment and rehabilitation may improve the patient situation and full thickness acute lesions have a potential to heal with repair tissue. This repair tissue, following acute lesions, can be compared to the repair following marrow stimulation and is not normal hyaline articular cartilage, but may function for smaller contained lesions.

Microfracture as a low cost minimally invasive procedure is preferred as the first-line cartilage repair technique on the medial/lateral femoral condyles and on the tibia. In my opinion, microfracture is not the best treatment for patellofemoral lesions. However, combining microfracture with a covering periosteum or membrane may be a better option. My first choice today, for lesions located on trochlea is ACI and on the patella I use microfracture covered by periosteum. Lesions on tibia needs often an extensive surgical approach for classic ACI surgery and microfracture is my first option for this location. Newer generations of ACI using cells in scaffolds that are delivered arthroscopically are promising in getting access to a more difficult area as the posterior tibia. It is also possible that aspects of ACI and microfracture may be combined in the same defect. ACI delivering in vitro grown cells and microfracture prepares a good bed for integration in addition to the elements from the bone marrow.

Patient having failed a microfracture procedure are good candidates for ACI. In some cases I do a re-microfracture especially for defects smaller than 4cm^2 considering the possibility that surgery and rehabilitation for the first procedure was not in line with recommended protocols. I believe that containment is important for a successful microfracture repair. The soft "super clot" is very vulnerable if not the defect has good surrounding cartilage shoulders. A recent study has reported an increased failure rate of ACI after previous treatment with marrow stimulation techniques[13]. The stiffening and violating of the subchondral bone plate may be important to avoid in larger non contained defects and can be used as an argument for trying ACI as a first line treatment in larger lesions.

Enhanced microfracture using a cover or scaffold to protect and/or soak up the cells may also be an option to ACI[14]. Growth factors and cytokines can be added to the repair site and gene therapy is also discussed[15].

The key question we soon need to answer: What is the role of the implanted cells (whether chondrocytes or stem cells) in the repair process? We are still lacking evidence from animal studies or long term clinical studies to be able to give a solid answer.

In addition to cartilage repair, joint instability and/or malalignment (Fig 2: ACI combined with HTO) should be addressed. Meniscus repair or even transplantation using allografts or scaffolds need to be considered. The safety profile of both ACI and microfracture has been acceptable and do not give us concern.

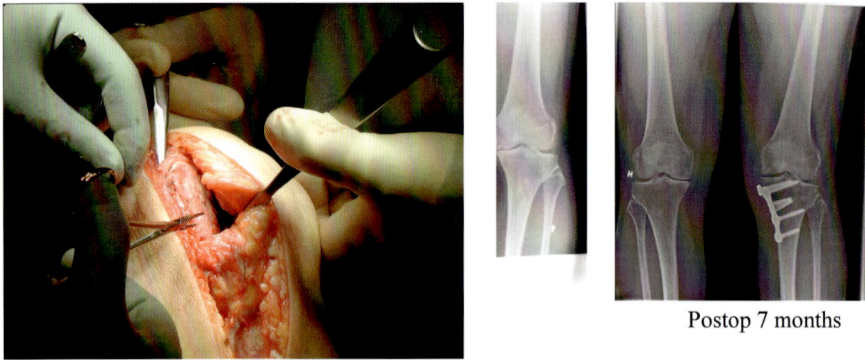

Postop 7 months

Figure 2: ACI combined with high tibial osteotomy. Large non contained defect on medial femoral condyle. Patient satisfied and improved 5 years after the operation.

Both ACI and microfracture have been used in other joints than the knee. The ankle joint is the second most frequent joint were isolated cartilage defects are treated surgically. Microfracture is my preferred first line treatment. Arthroscopy gives excellent access to this joint for the procedure. ACI represents an attractive salvage procedure for patients having failed microfracture and promising results have been published[16]. In many cases osteotomy of medial malleolus or distal fibula will be necessary for adequate surgical approach for classic ACI. In principle every joint in the upper or lower extremity are locations were cartilage repair may be applied. Cartilage repair procedures in shoulder, elbow and hip joint have been reported.

Conclusions

Both microfracture and ACI have documented satisfactory clinical outcome. Lack of randomised studies including non operative control groups is a major weakness. Long term studies should be performed to answer the question whether suboptimal cartilage tissue (fibrocartilage or mix hyaline-fibrocartilage) is a long lasting satisfactory solution for patients treated by biological repair techniques. In light of the available evidence today microfracture as a low cost and low morbidity procedure should be the preferred first line treatment for contained defects located on the medial/lateral femoral condyle and tibia. For defects larger than 4 cm^2 ACI or other procedures involving periosteum, membranes or scaffolds may be a better option. In my hands ACI is the preferred cartilage operation for trochlea defects needing resurfacing. For patients who microfracture has failed, ACI is a good option. It is generally accepted that the repair tissue following microfracture in adults do not represents native hyaline cartilage, therefore improvements for treatment of smaller (typical microfracture) defects are also needed. Some studies indicate that the structural repair following ACI has a more hyaline appearance, but what impact this has on long term clinical results has to be further evaluated. Enhanced microfracture techniques and newer genera-tions of ACI are promising and need further evaluations before any conclusions can be drawn. The enthusiastic and still increasing interest in the field of cartilage repair gives us hope for the years to come.

References

1. Brittberg M., Lindahl A, Nilsson A, Ohlsson C, Isaksson O, Peterson L: Treatment of deep cartilage defects in the knee with autologous chondrocyte transplantation. N Engl J Med 1994, 331: 889-895.

2. Steadman JR, Briggs KK, Rodrigo JJ, Kocher MS, Gill TJ, Rodkey WG: Outcomes of microfracture for traumatic chondral defects of the knee: Average 11-year follow-up. Arthroscopy 2003, 19: 477-484.

3. Knutsen G, Drogset J, Engebretsen L, Grontvedt T, Isaksen V, Ludvigsen T et al.: ACI v Microfracture - the picture at 5 years. In: Sports Knee Surgery 2005; 2005:193.

4. Knutsen G, Engebretsen L, Ludvigsen TC, Drogset JO, Grontvedt T, Solheim E et al.: Autologous chondrocyte implantation compared with microfracture in the knee. A randomized trial. J Bone Joint Surg Am 2004, 86-A: 455-464.

5. Bhosale AM, Richardson JB: Articular cartilage: structure, injuries and review of management. Br Med Bull 2008, 87: 77-95.

6. Brittberg M: Autologous chondrocyte implantation--technique and long-term follow-up. Injury 2008, 39 Suppl 1: S40-S49.

7. Jakobsen RB, Engebretsen L, Slauterbeck JR: An analysis of the quality of cartilage repair studies J Bone Joint Surg Am 2005, 87: 2232-2239.

8. Magnussen RA, Dunn WR, Carey JL, Spindler KP: Treatment of focal articular cartilage defects in the knee: a systematic review. Clin Orthop Relat Res 2008, 466: 952-962.

9. McNickle AG, Provencher MT, Cole BJ: Overview of existing cartilage repair technology. Sports Med Arthrosc 2008, 16: 196-201.

10. Pridie KH. A method for resurfacing the osteoarthritic knee joint. J.Bone Joint Surg.Br. 41, 618-619. 1959.

11. Wasiak J, Clar C, Villanueva E: Autologous cartilage implantation for full thickness articular carti-lage defects of the knee Cochrane Database Syst Rev 2006, 3: CD003323.

12. Saris DB, Vanlauwe J, Victor J, Haspl M, Bohnsack M, Fortems Y et al.: Characterized chondrocyte implantation results in better structural repair when treating symptomatic cartilage defects of the knee in a randomized controlled trial versus microfracture. Am J Sports Med 2008, 36: 235-246.

13. Minas T, Gomoll AH, Rosenberger R, Royce RO, Bryant T: Increased Failure Rate of Autologous Chondrocyte Implantation After Previous Treatment With Marrow Stimulation Techniques. Am J Sports Med 2009.

14. Kramer J, Bohrnsen F, Lindner U, Behrens P, Schlenke P, Rohwedel J: In vivo matrix-guided human mesenchymal stem cells Cell Mol Life Sci 2006, 63: 616-626.

15. Trippel S, Cucchiarini M, Madry H, Shi S, Wang C: Gene therapy for articular cartilage repair. Proc Inst Mech Eng [H] 2007, 221: 451-459.

16. Nam EK, Ferkel RD, Applegate GR: Autologous chondrocyte implantation of the ankle: a 2- to 5-year follow-up. Am J Sports Med 2009, 37: 274-284.

"The doctor has only one task: to cure the ill. The way he achieves it makes no difference"

(Hippocrates)

Chapter 16.

Bone Marrow Mesenchymal Stem Cells for Cartilage Repair

Konrad Slynarski, Jaroslaw Deszczynski

Take Home Message

Bone marrow is an easily available material with a potential for stimulating regeneration of the articular cartilage. Implanting bone marrow into the site of the chondral defect is a relatively easy procedure, which does not require additional manipulation outside the operating theatre, and makes it possible to obtain stable and lasting cartilage repair at the site of defect.

Introduction

The term mesenchymal stem cells (MSCs) signifies cells which can be harvested from bone marrow or other tissues and which are capable of differentiating into one or more types of connective tissue[2,3,6,16]. It is a heterogeneous group of cells which includes pluripotent stem cells capable of self-renewal and the progenitor cells developed out of them, which may be at different stages of development. Stem cells and progenitor cells are present in all the main tissues. In adults, stem cell populations are found practically in all organs. As an embryo develops into an adult, however, the capability of differentiating stem cells in each growing organ is gradually limited. During embryonic growth process, cells from the inner cell mass of the blastocyst retain the ability of complete regeneration and hence they are totipotent in terms of their differentiation potential. Yet, when the cells emerging out of those cells spread throughout the whole body and end up in appropriate tissues or organs, their differentiation potentiality is reduced.

The first formal presentation of the concept of pluripotent stem cells residing in the bone marrow can be found in Owen's publication[14]. In 1991, Caplan proposed the existence of mesenchymal stem cells (MSCs), capable of differentiating into a series of phenotypes of mesenchymal tissue[2]. According to this concept, a progenitor mesenchymal cell is able to differentiate toward bone, cartilage, muscle, elements of marrow, tendons and fatty tissue. This process requires that cell division take place, with a series of phenotype orientation and differentiation stages for the appropriate type of mesenchymal tissue. An attractive aspect of Caplan's hypothesis was that it provided for a possibility of manipulating these cells in order to bring about regeneration of destroyed tissue originating from this cell phenotype.

While the role of MSCs in the differentiation of tissues during the development process is well understood, the function that they should play in a mature individual remains the subject of discussion. It seems that a developing organism distributes progenitor cells in various tissues, with the intention of using them in potential future repair and reconstruction processes. One example confirming this concept are muscle satellite cells, located within the basement membrane of muscle fibres[9], which do not exhibit any protein expression unless activated to differentiate and undergo cell division[8]. MSCs in the bone marrow also function as a reservoir of pluripotent cells used in bone reconstruction following fracture or physiological bone reconstruction processes[7].

The role of MSCs in the bone marrow of adults may be as varied as the phenotypes presented by those cells. Whether MSCs perform this task directly, or through daughter cells – already differentiated progenitor cell pathways, restricted to individual phenotypes – is a question of the functioning of the progenitor cell system and the phenomenon of phenotypic plasticity of progenitor cells. Progenitor cells are present in a number of locations throughout the skeletal system. For example, the osteogenic and chondrogenic potential of the periosteum depends on the stem and progenitor cells located in its inner cambium layer[12,13]. These cells are also present in bone trabeculae and inside Haversian canals, as well as in fatty and muscle tissue[19]. Nevertheless, out of all the potential sources of progenitor cells the easiest and least invasive method involves harvesting them from the bone marrow by percutaneous biopsy. One potentially coherent theory explaining the presence of progenitor cells in fatty, muscle and other tissues is based on the presence in each of the above of pericytes, unique cells located outside the basement membrane of small blood vessels of all vascularised tissues. Pericytes isolated out of various tissues may, having been properly induced, be capable of differentiating into various connective tissue cells. In this way, it is suggested, pericytes may be representatives of the widespread generation of pluripotent cells.

The lifecycle of a stem or progenitor cell is a process regulated at five basic levels, i.e.: activation, proliferation, migration, differentiation and survival (or death). The activation of a progenitor cell from bone marrow is affected by EGF and PDGF. Whenever it occurs, more effective mitogens come into play: FGF-2, VEGF and moderate hypoxia[11].

144

Migration of progenitor cells is also made possible by the previously mentioned cytokines. It is presumed, however, that the modulators of its speed and direction may also be other factors: of chemotactic, bioactive and mechanical nature[5]. Differentiation of progenitor cells depends on the environment surrounding them. For example, bone marrow progenitor cells may develop into various cells, including into liver cells and central nervous system cells[15,17]. The most important early determinants influencing this process include partial pressure of oxygen, pH of the extracellular liquid, nutrient concentrations and factors of mechanical nature. The process is also affected by: the chemical composition of the surrounding extracellular liquid, contact with other cells as well as concentrations and gradients of various chemical signals (autocrine, paracrine and endocrine).

In addition, these MSCs secrete a variety of cytokines and growth factors that have both paracrine and autocrine functions. These secreted bioactive factors suppress the local immune system, inhibit fibrosis (scar formation) and apoptosis, enhance angiogenesis, as well as stimulate mitosis and differentiation of tissue-intrinsic reparative or stem cells. These effects, which are referred to as trophic effects, are distinct from the direct differentiation of MSCs into repair tissue[4].

This hypothesis is consistent with the concept presented in this chapter, of bone marrow implants as "information elements" serving to activate the repair processes in destroyed cartilage, and not just as a source of cells serving to rebuild the cartilage (however scarce a source).

Implanting fresh bone marrow into the chondral defect site

The procedure consists of a one-stage surgery, does not require further procedures outside the operating theatre and is performed using standard surgical instruments. The surgical technique used in implanting bone marrow resembles the classic technique for implanting chondrocytes as described by Brittberg et al. in 1994[1].

Apart from preparing the sterile field around the knee, one should also prepare a sterile field in the region of anterior iliac spine, so that it can be accessed during the procedure to perform the bone marrow biopsy.

The knee joint should be approached by mini- or open arthrotomy, depending on the location of the defect. After debriding the defect, measure it and prepare a template with aluminium foil, easily available in the operating theatre as a sterile suture packaging. During debridement, take care not to break subchondral bone or leave sharp perpendicular edges of the cartilage defect. According to the shape of the template, prepare a fragment of a commercially available collagen type I/III membrane patch matching the size of defect (Figure 1).

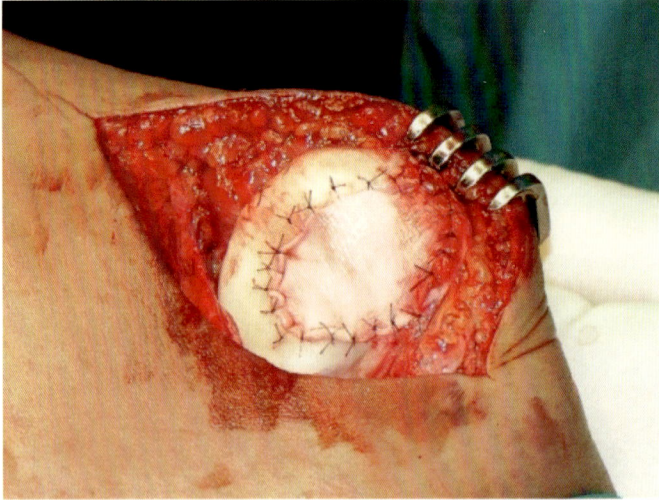

Figure 1: Collagen membrane covering cartilage defect.

The membrane should be inserted with the rough side towards the bone plate. The membrane is sutured with intermittent 5.0 absorbable sutures over the defect. Instead of collagen membrane, autologus periosteum harvested from upper medial part of tibia can be used (Figure 2).

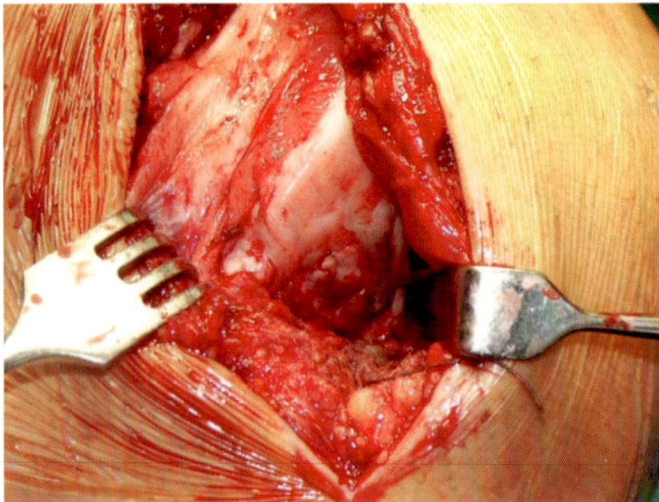

Figure 2: Periosteum covering the cartilage defect.

Periosteum can be harvested either from the supracondylar region of the femur or the medial region from the tibial tuberosity. Considering the smaller thickness and lower invasiveness during aspiration – the tibial region is recommended. The periosteum should be oriented with the cambium layer facing bone. Please note that the foil template is a mirror image of the defect, hence the membrane (or periosteum) should be cut out the right way, as if "looking down on the template lying upon the defect" (so that the rough side adheres to the bone). Then, anterior iliac crest should be punctured percutaneously with the aspirate needle, to harvest about 2 ml of bone marrow. Bone marrow must be implanted immediately under the membrane before it coagulates. The collagen membrane or periosteum can be additionally sealed with fibrin glue over the defect. This is not necessary, however, as the freshly harvested bone marrow coagulates under the membrane and the risk of leakage is low.

Bone marrow biopsy

A vital element in harvesting a good sample of bone marrow is the volume of the bone marrow aspirated. In order to obtain the most valuable specimen, I recommend that no more than 2 ml of bone marrow be aspirated from the ala of ilium. Normally, the chondral defect is small in volume and does not require more marrow. According to research published by Muschler[10], an increase in the aspiration volume from one to four millilitres caused a decrease of approximately 50 per cent in the final concentration of alkaline phosphatase-positive colony-forming units in an average sample. A larger volume decreases the concentration of progenitor cells because of the dilution of the sample with peripheral blood. If it is necessary to obtain larger quantities of bone marrow, for example in the case of multiple defects, it is recommended that a number of punctures of the ala of ilium be performed.

Rehabilitation

Immediately after the procedure, the limb is placed in a knee immobilizer. The following day (24 hours later), the patient starts range of movement exercise with the use of a continuous passive motion (CPM) splint, which is continued for approximately 6 weeks thereafter. The goal of rehabilitation is to achieve the full range of movement, gradual weight bearing by the operated limb and, ultimately, recovery of normal knee function.
In the case of defects localised on weight-bearing surfaces of the femoral condyle, the range of movement usually does not account for a problem and should reach about 90 degrees in the first few weeks. Gradual weight-bearing by the operated extremity, starting from approx. 20% of body weight can usually be commenced ca. 2-3 weeks after surgery and gradually increased while controlling the pain. Defects in the patellar-femoral joint require a period of limited bending up to approx. 40 degrees in the first 4-6 weeks, with weight-bearing up to the pain limit.

Usually, within 12-16 weeks patients regain the ability to perform everyday activities and stop using the orthosis. The following months, during which the implant undergoes a maturation process, require that exercise be performed in a way which does not interfere with the implant, while at the same time improving muscle strength and proprioception. Recommencing sports activity is usually permitted after about 12 months after surgery.

Complications

Bone marrow biopsy from the ala of ilium does not entail a significant risk of complications.

Apart from typical complications related to open knee surgery, there is a risk of periosteal graft hypertrophy, graft delamination and arthrofibrosis. Such complications, if diagnosed in time, usually permit a favourable prognosis. In the event of recurring pain, occurrence of exudate or locked knee, the joint should always be offloaded and an MRI exam done, preferably with a contrast agent (gadolinium) delivered intra-articularly. The next stage usually involves knee arthroscopy. Graft delamination typically involves only a part of the implant and usually the effective course of action is to debride the separated fragment and perform microfractures at the site. Although graft hypertrophy is a classic complication in periosteum implantations, yet collagen membrane grafts are not completely free of this risk (Figure 3 and 4).

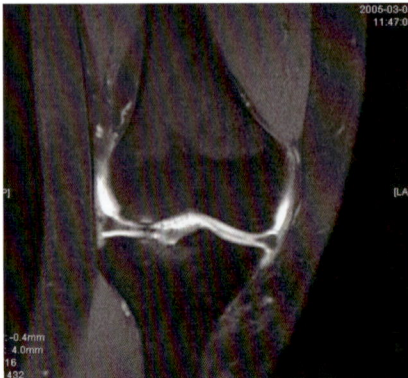

Figure 3: Graft hypertrophy of cartilage defect on lateral femoral condyle, treated with collagen membrane.

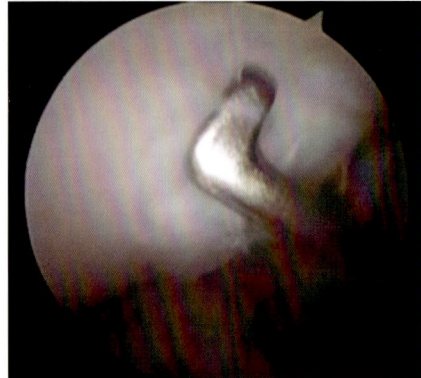

Figure 4: Arthroscopic appearance of hypertrophic membrane.

Most frequently, symptoms occur within 4-6 months after surgery and involve gradually increasing pain. Treatment involves gentle removal of excess tissue using arthroscopy down to the level of surrounding cartilage. Arthrofibroses usually occur more frequently in patients undergoing reconstruction in the patellar-femoral joint region. The emergence of adhesions may usually be suspected within the first few weeks after surgery and if despite increasing the intensity of rehabilitation exercise the adhesions do not subside in the first 3 months after surgery, arthroscopic lysis must be performed. In my experience, sometimes the graft can adhere to the synovial membrane and therefore I do not recommend lysis by manipulations under anaesthesia.

Discussion

Bone marrow grafts may be an effective alternative to other cell therapies in the treatment of articular cartilage defects. In the group of 14 patients with extensive chondral defects who underwent bone marrow and periosteum implants, at the 12-month follow-up nearly 86% of patients were classified as normal or nearly normal in the IKDC examination form[18]. MRI findings revealed surface with correct contour and continuity, without changes in subchondral bone in all but one patient. There was a positive correlation between the large size of defect, osteoarthritic nature of changes and poor results. In the histological assessment 2 years after implantation, good re-growth of cartilage was obtained as well as correct integration with the bone plate (Figure 5 and 6).

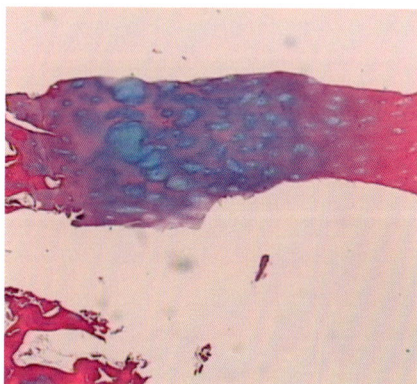

Figure 5: 53-year-old patient, 2 years after periosteum with bone marrow implantation.

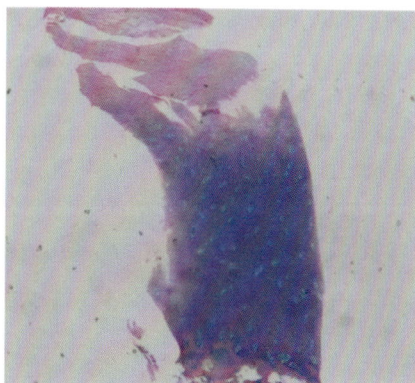

Figure 6: 25-year-old patient, 2 years after collagen membrane with bone marrow.

The hypothesis of bone marrow use is founded on the fact that it contains cells with a well-proven potential to differentiate into chondrocytes. Yet the ability to differentiate into the various phenotypes of mesenchymal cells is not the only way in which they can affect the regeneration process, because MSCs synthesize a broad spectrum of cytokines and growth factors. According to Caplan, the trophic effect of MSCs may be used in the treatment of cerebral stroke, cardiac infarction and meniscus repair[4]. Hence, bone marrow can be an advancement of the current strategies in tissue engineering based predominantly on cell grafts. It can be considered to be a type of "informative tissue" that supports local growth and differentiation of tissue. Of equal interest, from a similar point of view, is another element of this method – the periosteum. The advantage of using it is that it is at the same time a source of cells which can participate in cartilage repair, a way of delivering them and a natural scaffold, a mechanical barrier holding bone marrow in place and protecting the defect site as the regenerative tissue matures, and is a source of a series of growth factors regulating the functioning of chondrocytes and chondrogenesis[13]. These include transforming growth factor-beta 1, insulin-like growth factor-1, growth and differentiation factor-5, bone morphogenetic protein-2, integrins, and the receptors for these molecules. The method is based on the same hypothesis as microfractures and, in some sense, is an extension thereof. It, too, involves the presence of bone marrow at the site of chondral defect, except it takes place in a more controlled manner. It provides a stable scaffolding at the defect site, while at the same time creating a bioactive incubator, the active elements of which are bone marrow and periosteum. It is also important that this method of delivering bone marrow, unlike in the case of microfractures, does not interfere with the subchondral bone plate.

The use of periosteum, however, does entail certain risk of complications and requires an additional stage of the surgical procedure. It seems that periosteum can be effectively replaced with collagen membrane. The application of bone marrow coupled with periosteum or collagen membrane gives comparative results in goat models. Moreover, the surface layer of regenerated cartilage, when using a collagen membrane, is free of the fibrous top layer, which may lead to reducing the risk of periosteal graft hypertrophy and better durability of repaired tissue (Figure 7).

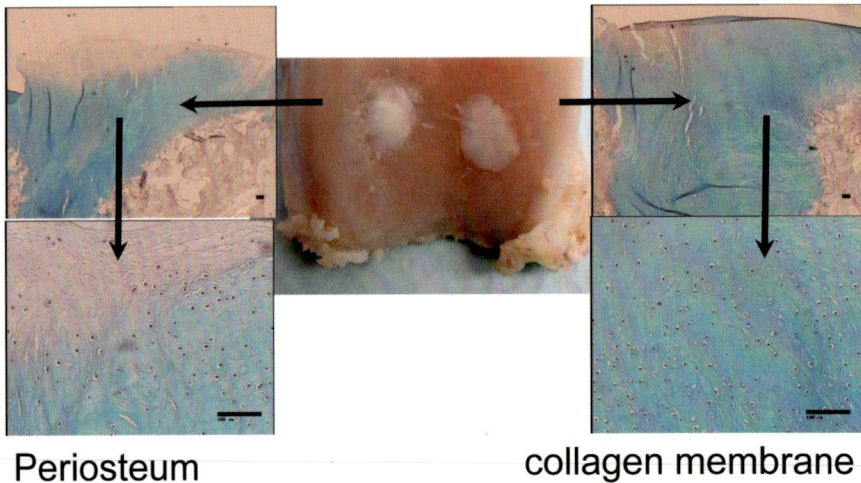

Periosteum   collagen membrane

Figure 7: Cartilage regeneration based on bone marrow and periosteum or collagen membrane on a goat model of two femoral defects on same animal.

References

1. Brittberg M., LindahlA, Nilsson A., Ohlsson C, Isaksson O., Peterson L: Treatment of deeo cartilage defects in the knee with autologous chondrocyte transplantation. N.Engl.J.Med.;331:889-895, 1994.
2. Caplan, Al. Mesenchymal stem cells. J Orthop Res;9:641–50, 1991
3. Caplan, Al. Embryonic development and the principles of tissue engineering. Novartis Found Symp 2003:249: 17-25; discussion 25-33, 170-4, 239-41.
4.Caplan Al, Dennis JE., Mesenchymal Stem Cells as Trophic Mediators. J Cell Biochem. 1;98(5):1076-84, 2006
5. de Crombrugghe, B., Lefebvre, V., Nakashima, K.; Regulatory mechanisms in the pathways of cartilage and bone formation, Curr.Op.Biol.,13:721-727, 2001
6. Friedenstein, A.J.; Precursors cells of mechanocytes. Int.Rev.Cytol. 47,327-359, 1976
7. Joyce, M.E., Jingushi, S., Scully, S.P., Bolander, M.E.; role of growth factors in fracture healing, Prog. Clin.Biol.Res.; 365;391-416. 1991
8. Lee KS, Kim HJ, Li QL, Chi XZ, Ueta C, Komori T, Wozney JM, Kim EG, Choi JY, Ryoo HM, Bae SC., Runx2 is a common target of transforming growth factor beta1 and bone morphogenetic protein 2, and co-operation between Runx2 and Smad5 induces osteoblast-specific gene expression in the pluripotent mesenchymal precursor cell line C2C12, Mol Cell Biol. ;20(23):8783-92. 2000
9. Mauro, A.; Satellite cell of skeletal muscle fibers, J Biophys Biochem Cytol.; 9:493 5. 1961
10. Muschler, GF, Boehm, C, Easley, K, Aspiration to obtain osteoblast progenitor cells from human bone marrow: the influence of aspiration volume., J Bone Joint Surg Am. 1997 Nov;79(11):1699-709.
11. Muschler, G.F., Midura, R.J.; Connective tissue progenitors: practical concepts for cinical applications, Clin.Orthop.Rel.Res., 395, 66-80, 2002
12. Nakahara, H., Goldberg, V.M., Caplan, A.I.;Culture-expanded human periosteal-derived cells exhibit osteochondral potential in vivo, J.Orthop.Res, 9:465-476, 1991
13. O'Driscoll, S.W., Fitzsimmons, J.S.; The role of periosteum in cartilage repair, Clin.Orthop.Rel. Res.,391S, S190-S207, 2001
14. Owen M.; Marrow stromal stem cells, J Cell Sci Suppl.;10:63-76. 1988
15. Petersen, B.E., Bowen, W.C., Patrene, K.D., i wsp.; Bone marrow as a potential source of hepatic oval cells, Science 284, 1168-1170, 1999
16. Pittenger, M.F., Mackay, A.M., Beck, S.C., Jaiswal, R.K., Douglas, R., Mosca, J.D., Moorman, M.A., Simonetti, D.W., Craig, S., Marshak, D.R.; Multilineage potential of adult mesenchymal stem cells, Science, 284, 143-147, 1999
17. Rao, M.S., Multipotent and restricted precursors in the central nervous system. Anat.Rec., 257:137-148, 1999
18. Slynarski, K., Deszczynski, J., Karpinski J.; Fresh bone marrow and periosteum transplantation for cartilage defects of the knee, Transplant Proc.;38(1):318-919. 2006 Toriyama, K., Kawaguchi, N., Kitoh, J., Rie Tajma, M.A., Inou, K., Kitagawa, Y., Torii, S.; Endogenous adipocyte precursor cells for regenerative soft-tissue engineering, T.Eng. 8, 1, 157-164, 2002

Acknowledgments

The author of this chapter wishes to thank Dr Sebastian Concaro from the Department of Orthopaedics and Department of Molecular Biology and Regenerative Medicine, Sahlgrenska University Hospital, Gothenburg, Sweden for his assistance with histological evaluation.

"The most exciting phrase to hear in science, the one that heralds the most discoveries, is not "Eureka!" (I found it!) but "That's funny..."

(Isaac Asimov)

Chapter 17.

Magnetic Resonance Imaging of Cartilage Repair

Stefan Marlovits, Goetz Welsch, Siegfried Trattnig

Take home message

Cartilage repair techniques require a noninvasive standardized and high quality follow-up to assess the structure of repair tissue, a goal that is best fulfilled by Magnetic Resonance Imaging (MRI).
Standard morphological MR evaluation of cartilage repair tissue can be performed using the same acquisition techniques as those used for native cartilage or in OA.
The perhaps most complete MR evaluation is performed by the magnetic resonance observation of cartilage repair tissue (MOCART) scoring system.

Introduction

Articular cartilage injuries and degenerative joint diseases are very common and affect a significant proportion of the population of all ages[1]. Many patients may benefit from cartilage repair surgeries which can offer the chance to avoid the development of osteoarthritis or delay its progression. Over the past decade, a number of surgical interventions have been developed in the attempt to produce a durable repair[2-3]. These methods may be arthroscopic or open surgical techniques, and include marrow-stimulation techniques, such as drilling and microfracture, osteochondral grafts, periosteal or perichondral grafts, and autologous chondrocyte implantation (ACT) using a periosteal flap or the combination of biomaterials with chondrocytes as a matrix-based cell implantation (MACI)[4]. Cartilage repair techniques require a noninvasive standardized and high quality follow-up to assess the structure of repair tissue, a goal that is best fulfilled by Magnetic Resonance Imaging (MRI).

MRI is the method of choice for the evaluation of articular cartilage. With MRI, a powerful tool for the non-invasive visualization of articular cartilage and the monitoring of articular cartilage degeneration and regeneration in vivo is available[5]. The use of cartilage-sensitive sequences and high spatial resolution techniques allow accurate evaluation of cartilage morphology, even in the earlier stages of disease, as well as an analysis of cartilage repair tissue during follow-up. With the use of appropriate techniques, it is possible to evaluate the biochemical and biomechanical status of cartilage in addition to cartilage morphology. These benefits make MRI a useful tool for the initial diagnosis and subsequent postoperative monitoring of cartilage lesions and cartilage repair tissue.

Basic MR technical requirements

Magnetic resonance imaging is a non-invasive, non-contact, multi-planar technique capable of producing high resolution, high contrast images in serial contiguous slices. Native articular cartilage and postoperative cartilage repair tissue are relatively thin structures that cover curved surfaces and thus require high quality, high resolution images for accurate assessment. MRI techniques allows morphological assessment of the cartilage surface, thickness, volume, and subchondral bone[6-11]. In addition, MRI techniques can be used to evaluate the biochemical and biomechanical status of articular cartilage. MRI of cartilage and cartilage repair can be obtained at most clinically available MR systems. It has been demonstrated that a voxel size under 300µm is required to reveal fraying of the articular surface of cartilage[12]. The introduction of high field MRI units with 1.5 T and especially 3.0 T has provided the means to achieve such resolution while maintaining reasonable scan times using cartilage-sensitive sequences. High field MRI also increases the possibilities for three-dimensional (3D) acquisitions yielding high resolution and high signal- and contrast-to-noise ratio. Furthermore isotropic MRI and its multiplanar reconstruction (MPR) provides the possibility to image the repair tissue in every reformatted plane without any loss of resolution[9,13-14].

Cartilage specific sequences

Standard morphological MR evaluation of cartilage repair tissue can be performed using the same acquisition techniques as those used for native cartilage or in OA[5]. The most commonly used MR imaging techniques are intermediate-weighted, fast spin-echo (FSE) with or without fat-suppression and three-dimensional (3D) fat-suppressed gradient-echo (GRE) acquisitions[5-7,10,15]. Whereas the GRE sequence visualizes cartilage defects attributable to T1 differences between cartilage and fluid, the FSE sequence uses differences in T2 weighting.

Fast spin echo (FSE) imaging combines the heavy T2 weighting, magnetization transfer effects, and relative preservation of high signal intensity in the marrow fat to produce subchondral bone that exhibits a high signal intensity. Thus, this technique exploits dark cartilage against bright synovial fluid with consecutive high contrast between cartilage and adjacent joint fluid and bone marrow[16-17] (Fig 1).

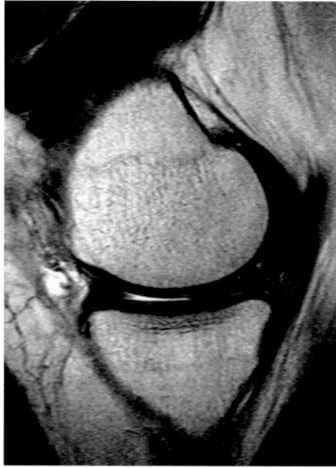

Figure 1: Sagittal T2-FSE image of the knee joint, with dark cartilage against bright synovial fluid.

Collagen fibers with a highly regular structure, particularly near the cartilage-bone interface, tend to immobilize water molecules and promote dipolar interactions between their protons, thus accelerating T2 relaxation. T2-weighted FSE sequences are, therefore, useful for both the detection of surface and matrix damage assessed by intrachondral signal abnormalities. The T2-weighted FSE sequence is relatively insensitive to magnetic susceptibility artifacts, which is advantageous in patients who have undergone previous surgery of the joint.

The advantage of fat-suppressed 3D gradient echo sequences is the relatively high signal intensity of articular cartilage in contrast to low signal intensity from the adjacent fat-suppressed tissue (Fig 2)

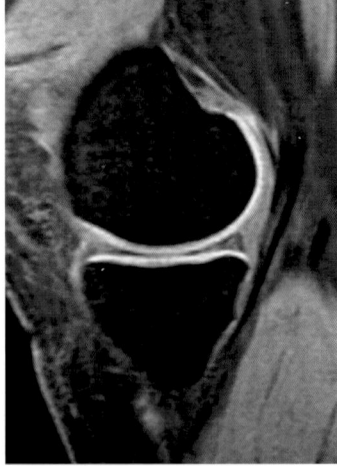

Figure 2: Sagittal T1-weighted, 3D, GRE image of the knee joint, with bright carti-lage signal against low signal from the adjacent fat-suppressed tissue.

Three-dimensional acquisitions yield images with higher out-of-plane resolution and contrast-to-noise ratio than two-dimensional acquisitions. Fat-suppressed, 3D gradient echo imaging is easy to perform and is widely available[6-8,11,14]. The 3D data set can be used for reformatting in any plane and for 3D visualization and volume measurements[6,12,14]. Both sequences, the fat-suppressed 3D GRE and the T2-weighted FSE, are showing excellent results with high sensitivity, specificity and accuracy for detecting cartilage lesions in the knee[5,13].

Morphological MRI and classification systems

Different MRI classification systems have been used to describe articular cartilage changes[15,18]. For the description of the morphology of the repair the repair tissue is compared to the adjacent native cartilage. On MR images, the repair tissue should ideally appear as thick as the adjacent native cartilage, and should have a smooth articular surface that reproduces the original articular contour[19]. The signal intensity of the repair tissue should be isointense to the adjacent native cartilage. The variables of pathological changes in hyaline cartilage and cartilage defects include altered tissue signal intensity, abnormal surface contour, and changes in cartilage thickness and volume[20]. For the use of MRI in the evaluation of cartilage repair techniques an evaluation system that has low interobserver variability and is suited for statistical data analysis is necessary. It should have the potential to compare different cartilage surgery techniques and also to be used in multi-center studies[21-22]. Although fat-suppressed, 3D, gradient-echo images are more useful for assessing contour defects, FSE images are more useful for assessing intrachondral signal abnormalities[10]. Only if sufficient joint effusion is present can contour defects be evaluated accurately with FSE sequences (Fig 3).

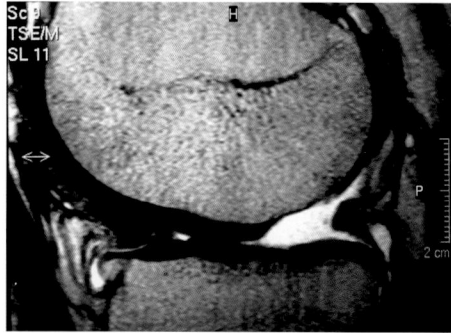

Figure 3: Sagittal T2-FSE image of the knee joint, with a full-thickness cartilage defect in the medial femoral condyle.

Thus, the combination of both sequences should be used to assess cartilage defects[15]. This can be done without significant compromise in terms of imaging time or the accurate assessment of derangements other than cartilage lesions[15]. The most commonly used MRI classification system of chondral lesions is based on the classification of Yulish et al.[18]. In this grading system, four different grades, with respect to intrachondral signal abnormalities and the depth of cartilage defects, are used (Table 1). In addition to this grading scheme, the size and location of a lesion should be evaluated and described[20].

Grade 1	Abnormal intrachondral signal with a normal chondral surface
Grade 2	Mild surface irregularity and/or focal loss of less than 50% of the cartilage thickness
Grade 3	Severe surface irregularity with focal loss of 50% to 100% of the cartilage thickness
Grade 4	Complete loss of articular cartilage, with exposure of subchondral bone

Table 1: MRI classification of articular chondral lesions[18].

When choosing the image acquisition protocol for a particular patient after surgical cartilage repair, it is important to know the type of cartilage repair performed, size and location within the joint, and concomitant procedures, such as osteotomy or ligament repair (Fig. 4).

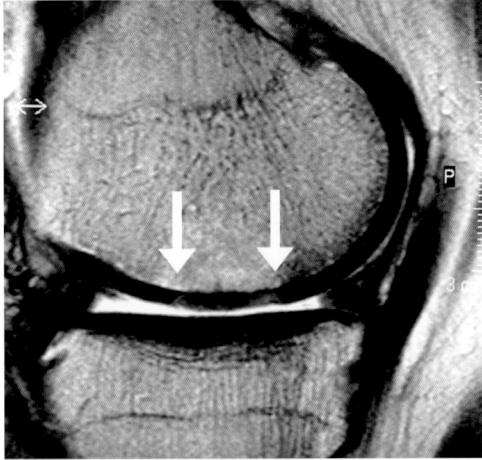

Figure 4: Cartilage repair tissue 12 months after matrix-associated autologous chondrocyte transplantation (MACT) with ideal morphology: complete filling of the defect and complete integration to the adjacent cartilage and subchondral bone with a smooth surface and no changes in the subchondral bone plate (high resolution sagittal T2-FSE image; arrows indicates the cartilage repair tissue).

A few different classification systems for the description of articular cartilage repair tissue have been proposed[21-22]. But, for optimal use, a simple evaluation and a point scoring system that allows efficient statistical data analysis is necessary. Roberts et al. used four parameters to assess cartilage repair on MR images: surface integrity and contour; cartilage signal in the graft region; cartilage thickness; and changes in underlying bone[22]. A score is obtained by summing the values of the four parameters; scores range from 0 (no repair) to a maximum of 4 (complete repair). Unfortunately, the system only assesses each parameter as normal or abnormal, and provides no assessment of the graft integration, degree of defect fill, or the presence of adhesions. The perhaps most complete MR evaluation is performed by the magnetic resonance observation of cartilage repair tissue (MOCART) scoring system (Table 2)[21, 23].

Variables

1. Degree of defect repair and filling of the
    complete
    hypertrophy
    incomplete
        >50% of the adjacent cartilage
        <50% of the adjacent cartilage
        subchondral bone exposed

2. Integration to border zone
    complete
    incomplete
        demarcating border visible (split-like)
        defect visible: <50% of the length of the repair tissue
                    >50% of the length of the repair tissue

3. Surface of the repair tissue
    surface intact
    surface damaged
        <50% of repair tissue depth
        >50% of repair tissue depth or total degeneration

4. Structure of the repair tissue
    homogenous
    inhomogeneous or cleft formation

5. Signal intensity of the repair tissue
    Dual T2-FSE
        isointense
        moderately hyperintense
        markedly hyperintense
    3D-GE-FS
        isointense
        moderately hypointense
        markedly hypointense

6. Subchondral Lamina
    intact
    not intact

7. Subchondral bone
    intact
    not intact

8. Ahesions
    no
    yes

9. Effusion
    no
    yes

Table 2: MRI classification of articular cartilage repair tissue[21]
MOCART (Magentic Resonance Observation of CArtilage Repair Tissue).

Based on the possibilities of MPR of an isotropic MR dataset a new 3D MOCART score was recently introduced and compared to the standard 2D MOCART with high correlation of the single variables (Table 3)[24].

	Variables	
1.	**Defect fill** 0 % 0-25 % 25-50 % 50-75 % 75-100 % 100 % 100-125 % 125-150 % 150-200% > 200%	
2.	**Cartilage interface** Complete Sagittal (Femur, Patella, Trochlea, Tibia) Demarcating border visible Defect visible <50% Defect visible >50%	Complete Coronal (Femur, Tibia), Axial (Patella, Trochlea) Demarcating border visible Defect visible <50% Defect visible >50%
3.	**Bone interface** Complete Partial delamination Complete delamination Delamination of periosteal flap	
4.	**Surface** Intact Surface demaged <50% depth Surface demaged >50% depth Adhesions	
5.	**Structue** Homogenous Inhomogenous or Cleft formation	
6.	**Signal Intensity** Normal (identical to adjacent cartilage) Nearly normal (slight areas of signal alteration) Abnormal (large areas of signal alteration)	
7.	**Subchondral lamina** Intact Not intact	
8.	**Chondral Osteophytes** Absent Osteophyt with thickness <0,25 cm Osteophyt with thickness >0,25 cm	
9.	**Bone marrow edema** Absent Small (<1cm) Medium (<2cm) Large (<4cm) Diffuse	
10.	**Subchondral bone** Intact Not intact (Granulation tissue, cyst, sclerosis)	
11.	**Effusion** Absent Small Medium Large **Max**	

Table 3: MRI classification of articular cartilage repair tissue[24]
3D MOCART (Magentic Resonance Observation of CArtilage Repair Tissue).

The different variables are defect fill (1), cartilage interface (2), bone interface (3), surface of the repair tissue (4), structure of the repair tissue (5), signal intensity of the repair tissue (6), subchondral lamina (7), chondral osteophyte (8), bone marrow edema (9), subchondral bone (10) and effusion (11)[24].

Functional (biochemical) MRI

a) dGEMRIC for the assessment of cartilage repair

T1 relaxation enhanced by delayed administration of gadolinium diethylenetriamine pentaacetate anion (Gd-DTPA2-) the dGEMRIC (delayed Gadolinium enhanced MRI of cartilage) technique, is currently the most widely used method for analyzing proteoglycan depletion in articular cartilage and has provided valuable results in vitro and in vivo. Glycosaminoglycans (GAG), with their negatively charged side chains, are the main source of fixed charge density (FCD) in cartilage, which are thought to be the first component of the extracellular matrix to be lost in early cartilage degeneration. Intravenously administered gadolinium diethylenetriamine pentaacetate anion (Gd-DTPA2-) penetrates the cartilage through both the articular surface and the subchondral bone and the negative contrast equilibrates in inverse relation to the FCD, which is, in turn, directly related to the GAG concentration. Therefore, T1, which is determined by the Gd-DTPA2- concentration, becomes a specific measure of tissue GAG concentration. T1 relaxation enhanced by delayed administration of Gd-DTPA2-, the dGEMRIC (delayed Gadolinium Enhanced MRI of Cartilage) technique, can be considered the method of choice for detecting proteoglycan depletion in articular cartilage[25-27] (Fig. 5).

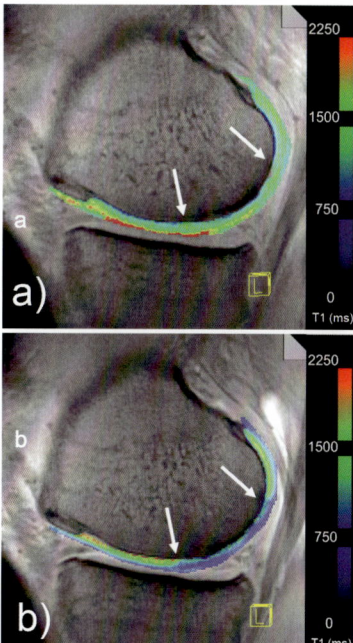

Figure 5: Biochemical sagittal T1 dGEMRIC images of a patient after MACT (same as Fig. 6) of the medial femoral condyle (arrows). Whereas a) is showing pre-contrast fused T1 map, b) is showing the same plane for the post-contrast evaluation. For quantitative T1 mapping a GRE sequence (15/3.15; flip angles 4.4° and 24.7°) with high resolution (448x448; 16cm; slice thickness 3mm) and 16 slides applied in 3:40 minutes.

In dGEMRIC experiments, T1-mapping is performed. An increased accumulation of contrast agent due to a focal depletion of GAG results in lower T1 values in this degenerative cartilage region compared to healthy cartilage. T1 is high in normal cartilage and low in GAG-depleted, osteoarthritic cartilage. For post-contrast MR imaging the dGEMRIC protocol proposed by Burstein et al.[27] is used, i.e., application of a bolus of 0.2mmol contrast agent per kilogram body weight (double dose). After injection, the patient should be subjected to moderate exercise of the knee by walking up and down stairs for about twenty minutes. Ninety minutes after contrast-application the post-contrast MR imaging should be performed, to allow for sufficient time for the contrast agent (Gd) to diffuse into the cartilage layer before the images are acquired.

b) Quantitative MR T1 rho
T1 rho-weighted MR imaging or spin-lattice relaxation in the rotating frame is a time constant that defines the relaxation of spins under the influence of the radiofrequency (RF) field T1 rho. T1 rho has been correlated to fixed charge density in both enzymatically-degraded bovine and human osteoarthritic explants, where normalized T1 rho rate was strongly correlated to alterations in fixed charge density due to depletion of proteoglycan, as confirmed by histology[28].

c) T2 mapping
T2 mapping and other techniques that assess collagen provide complimentary information to those techniques targeted to proteoglycan[29-30] (Fig 6).

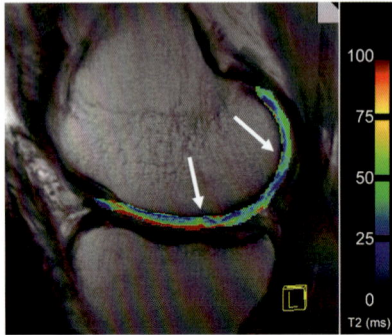

Figure 6: Sagittal multi-echo spin-echo T2 (1200/12.9, 25.8, 38.7, 51.6, 65.5, 77.4; flip angle 180°) sequence with high inplane resolution (384 x 384; 16cm; 3mm slice thickness) visualizing a patient 60 months after MACT (arrows) within the medial femoral condyle of the knee (same patient as figure 3). 12 slices were achieved for T2 in 4:37 minutes.

In vitro T2 relaxation studies revealed a close relation of T2 to the architecture of collagen[31-32]. Quantitative T2 mapping has been shown at both high field and clinically relevant field strengths to correlate to collagen orientation[33-34]. Thus, a major contribution from collagen orientation and collagen concentration to the T2 value is important. In acquiring T2 maps of articular cartilage, classically, a multi-echo spin-echo sequence is used, followed by T2 map calculation with a non-linear fitting algorithm. Several investigators have measured the spatial distribution of T2 relaxation times within cartilage. In native hyaline cartilage, there is a depth-wise variation of T2 relaxation times with shorter T2 values in the radial zone, where the collagen is highly ordered, and longer values in the transitional zone due to less organization of the collagen. The spatial distribution of the T2 relaxation time can be used for in vivo monitoring of the biomechanical properties of various cartilage layers, pathological changes, or aging[35-36].

References

1. Elders, M.J., The increasing impact of arthritis on public health. J Rheumatol Suppl, 2000. 60: p. 6-8.
2. Jackson, D.W., M.J. Scheer, and T.M. Simon, Cartilage substitutes: overview of basic science and treatment options. J Am Acad Orthop Surg, 2001. 9(1): p. 37-52.
3. Simon, T.M. and D.W. Jackson, Articular cartilage: injury pathways and treatment options. Sports Med Arthrosc, 2006. 14(3): p. 146-54.
4. Hunziker, E.B., Articular cartilage repair: basic science and clinical progress. A review of the current status and prospects. Osteoarthritis Cartilage, 2002. 10(6): p. 432-63.
5. Recht, M., et al., Magnetic resonance imaging of articular cartilage. Clin Orthop Relat Res, 2001(391 Suppl): p. S379-96.
6. Disler, D.G., Fat-suppressed three-dimensional spoiled gradient-recalled MR imaging: assessment of articular and physeal hyaline cartilage. AJR Am J Roentgenol, 1997. 169(4): p. 1117-23.
7. Kawahara, Y., et al., Fast spin-echo MR of the articular cartilage in the osteoarthrotic knee. Correlation of MR and arthroscopic findings. Acta Radiol, 1998. 39(2): p. 120-5.
8. Peterfy, C.G., et al., MR imaging of the arthritic knee: improved discrimination of cartilage, synovium, and effusion with pulsed saturation transfer and fat-suppressed T1-weighted sequences. Radiology, 1994. 191(2): p. 413-9.
9. Peterfy, C.G., et al., Quantification of the volume of articular cartilage in the metacarpophalangeal joints of the hand: accuracy and precision of three-dimensional MR imaging. AJR Am J Roentgenol, 1995. 165(2): p. 371-5.
10. Potter, H.G., et al., Magnetic resonance imaging of articular cartilage in the knee. An evaluation with use of fast-spin-echo imaging. J Bone Joint Surg Am, 1998. 80(9): p. 1276-84.
11. Trattnig, S., et al., Imaging articular cartilage defects with 3D fat-suppressed echo planar imaging: comparison with conventional 3D fat-suppressed gradient echo sequence and correlation with histology. J Comput Assist Tomogr, 1998. 22(1): p. 8-14.
12. Rubenstein, J.D., et al., Image resolution and signal-to-noise ratio requirements for MR imaging of degenerative cartilage. AJR Am J Roentgenol, 1997. 169(4): p. 1089-96.
13. Disler, D.G., et al., Fat-suppressed three-dimensional spoiled gradient-echo MR imaging of hyaline cartilage defects in the knee: comparison with standard MR imaging and arthroscopy. AJR Am J Roentgenol, 1996. 167(1): p. 127-32.
14. Recht, M.P., et al., Accuracy of fat-suppressed three-dimensional spoiled gradient-echo FLASH MR imaging in the detection of patellofemoral articular cartilage abnormalities. Radiology, 1996. 198(1): p. 209-12.
15. Trattnig, S., et al., Magnetic resonance imaging of articular cartilage and evaluation of cartilage disease. Invest Radiol, 2000. 35(10): p. 595-601.
16. Constable, R.T., et al., Factors influencing contrast in fast spin-echo MR imaging. Magn Reson Imaging, 1992. 10(4): p. 497-511.

17. Yao, L., A. Gentili, and A. Thomas, Incidental magnetization transfer contrast in fast spin-echo imaging of cartilage. J Magn Reson Imaging, 1996. 6(1): p. 180-4.

18. Yulish, B.S., et al., Chondromalacia patellae: assessment with MR imaging. Radiology, 1987. 164(3): p. 763-6.

19. Alparslan, L., et al., Postoperative magnetic resonance imaging of articular cartilage repair. Semin Musculoskelet Radiol, 2001. 5(4): p. 345-63.

20. Recht, M.P., et al., Abnormalities of articular cartilage in the knee: analysis of available MR techniques. Radiology, 1993. 187(2): p. 473-8.

21. Marlovits, S., et al., Definition of pertinent parameters for the evaluation of articular cartilage repair tissue with high-resolution magnetic resonance imaging. Eur J Radiol, 2004. 52(3): p. 310-9.

22. Roberts, S., et al., Autologous chondrocyte implantation for cartilage repair: monitoring its success by magnetic resonance imaging and histology. Arthritis Res Ther, 2003. 5(1): p. R60-73.

23. Marlovits, S., et al., Magnetic resonance observation of cartilage repair tissue (MOCART) for the evaluation of autologous chondrocyte transplantation: determination of interobserver variability and correlation to clinical outcome after 2 years. Eur J Radiol, 2006. 57(1): p. 16-23.

24. Welsch, G.H., et al., Three-dimensional magnetic resonance observation of cartilage repair tissue (MOCART) score assessed with an isotropic three-dimensional true fast imaging with steady-state precession sequence at 3.0 Tesla. Invest Radiol, 2009. 44(9): p. 603-12.

25. Bashir, A., M.L. Gray, and D. Burstein, Gd-DTPA2- as a measure of cartilage degradation. Magn Reson Med, 1996. 36(5): p. 665-73.

26. Bashir, A., et al., Nondestructive imaging of human cartilage glycosaminoglycan concentration by MRI. Magn Reson Med, 1999. 41(5): p. 857-65.

27. Burstein, D., et al., Protocol issues for delayed Gd(DTPA)(2-)-enhanced MRI (dGEMRIC) for clinical evaluation of articular cartilage. Magn Reson Med, 2001. 45(1): p. 36-41.

28. Wheaton, A.J., et al., Correlation of T1rho with fixed charge density in cartilage. J Magn Reson Imaging, 2004. 20(3): p. 519-25.

29. Domayer, S.E., et al., T2 mapping and dGEMRIC after autologous chondrocyte implantation with a fibrin-based scaffold in the knee: Preliminary results. Eur J Radiol, 2009.

30. Potter, H.G. and L.F. Foo, Magnetic resonance imaging of articular cartilage: trauma, degeneration, and repair. Am J Sports Med, 2006. 34(4): p. 661-77.

31. Menezes, N.M., et al., T2 and T1rho MRI in articular cartilage systems. Magn Reson Med, 2004. 51(3): p. 503-9.

32. Nieminen, M.T., et al., T2 relaxation reveals spatial collagen architecture in articular cartilage: a comparative quantitative MRI and polarized light microscopic study. Magn Reson Med, 2001. 46(3): p. 487-93.

33. Xia, Y., Heterogeneity of cartilage laminae in MR imaging. J Magn Reson Imaging, 2000. 11(6): p. 686-93.

34. White, L.M., et al., Cartilage T2 assessment: differentiation of normal hyaline cartilage and reparative tissue after arthroscopic cartilage repair in equine subjects. Radiology, 2006. 241(2): p. 407-14.

35. Smith, H.E., et al., Spatial variation in cartilage T2 of the knee. J Magn Reson Imaging, 2001. 14(1): p. 50-5.

36. Mosher, T.J., B.J. Dardzinski, and M.B. Smith, Human articular cartilage: influence of aging and early symptomatic degeneration on the spatial variation of T2--preliminary findings at 3 T. Radiology, 2000. 214(1): p. 259-66.

37. Kaufman, J.H., et al., A novel approach to observing articular cartilage deformation in vitro via magnetic resonance imaging. J Magn Reson Imaging, 1999. 9(5): p. 653-62.

"In re-operative surgery, timing is everything"

(Timothy Fabian)

Chapter 18.

Failed Articular Cartilage Repair: What To Do?

Mats Brittberg

Take Home Message

Remember to look at potential causes of a cartilage repair failure:
- *Non-committed patient*
- *Overweight*
- *Smoking*
- *Instability*
- *Malalignement*
- *Other diseases such as diabetes and similar endocrine diseases*
- *The subchondral bone appearance - hard bone or soft bone*
- *Quality of surrounding cartilage*

Summarize and make a rescue plan. Take your time to plan. Cartilage repair is a very slow process. You do not need to hurry.

Introduction

The main indication for cartilage repair is pain in rest, pain in motions and followed by degrees of mechanical symptoms. Small lesions that are partial thickness defects grade ICRS I-II may be treated by debridement while deeper lesions from ICRS Grade III to IV need a more aggressive treatment plan[4]. For small to medium sized defects, most often microfracture technique is used today[4]. For larger

165

defects, autologous chondrocyte implantation, mosaicplasty and allografts are potential options[4]. Recently, newer one-stage procedures such as OBI trufit[5], CAIS[11] and Maioregen[9] have been introduced to the market.
However, how to do when our primary cartilage repair technique fails?

The rescue plan

I believe it is mandatory to follow a rescue plan with the following components:
1. New plain x-rays with long alignment evaluation-HKA
2. MRI to study the subchondral bone. There may also be a need for a complimentory isotope scan.
3. New assessment arthroscopy.
4. Re-analyze the postoperative rehabilitation that the patient has had or has not followed strictly.
5. If the patient is a smoker, try to get the patient to quit smoking.
6. If the patient is over weight, induce weight reducing therapy.

Femoral Condyles

If the patient has a very large condylar defect, but no malalignment, consider unloading osteotomy for your next surgery or unloading brace postoperatively
When a large defect is seen in a patient with malignment; combine new repair with unloading osteotomy (preferably opening wedge).

Patellar defects

Patellar defects may be influenced by patellar instability and the patellofemoral joints need a very careful re-evaluation preoperatively.
The patella will be articulating on more proximal cartilage with the knee flexed.
Proximal patellar lesion responds poorly to tibial tubercle anteriorization procedures as such an operation causes load shift onto more proximal patella[6].
An overly medialized tibial tubercle with a painful and poorly repaired cartilage patellar lesion may need to be returned to a lateral position via an anterolateral tibial tubercle transfer, re-routing of the patella[6].
Lateral release will relieve abnormal tilt of the patella but if there is lateral facet degeneration also osteotomy is needed; an anteromedial tib.tubercle transfer[6,13].
Medialization may cause too much medial loading. Be careful when to treat medial lesions! Hauser plasty as it is a posteromedial transfer could cause medial patellar cartilage breakdown[6]!!

Which technique to use ?

If one believes that the repair with bone marrow stimulation was not done properly, a second repeat microfracture may be performed if the lesion is small (<2 cm²). Otherwise, one may choose other cartilage repair technologies.

As up to date, no methods have been shown to be better than other, the choice is free. However, one should evaluate a possible increased stiffness of the subchondral bone with sclerotic bone and less number of vessels.

If one consider to choose to do a second bone marrow stimulation one may use subchondral drilling instead of microfracture while drilling gets assess to larger vessels and by that increased chance of stronger ingrowth of mesenchymal stem cells.

However, for large defects one has to cover large surfaces and methods with different cell-seeded scaffolds are subsequently more interesting for use. If the subchondral bone is involved concommittant bone grafting may be needed or use of a technique that directly involves also the bone such as mosaicplasty with autografts, OBI Trufit[5] or Maioregen[9].

Examples of different partially or totally failed cartilage repairs

A partially insufficient microfracture repair may be augmented with implantation of carbon fibre rods[3]. (Fig 1)

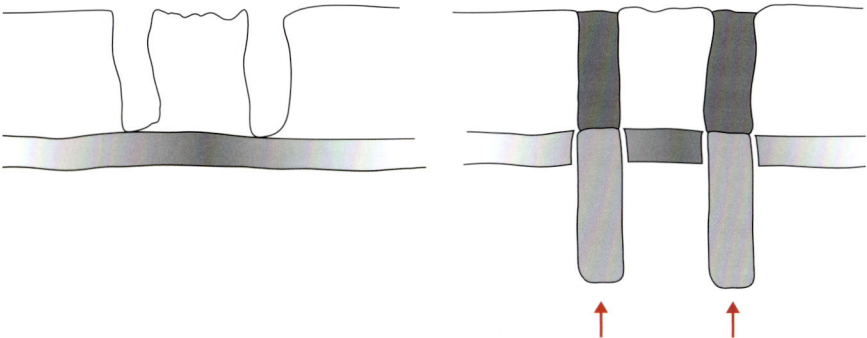

Figure 1: A partially insufficient microfracture repair may be augmented with implantation of carbon fibre rods. The ingrowing strong fibrocartilaginous tissue gives support to the intial repair.

A partially failed ACI with border insufficiency may also be treated by border zone implantation with carbon rods.

A failed carbon fibre rod implanted area may be substituted by an OBI Trufit plug also taken care of the bone region or an autologous mosaic plug.

A failed first generation ACI (Periost + cells) may be restituted by a third generation ACI such as Hyalograft14, MACI1 or similar.

167

Failures of osteochondral repair

Failed mosaicplasty may be operated on with 3rd gen. ACI + bone grafting as one-stage.

The choice of how to treat a failed subchondral repair depends on the earlier method that has been used.

Small to medium sized defects can be treated by implantation of autologous osteochondral plugs (Fig.1.) solving both the osseous and cartilaginous loss of tissue[7] (Fig 2).

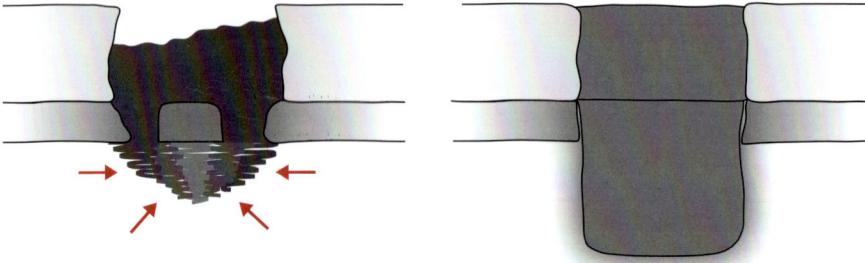

Figure 2: Small to medium sized osteochondral defects can be treated by implantation of autologous osteochondral plugs solving both the osseous and cartilaginous loss of tissue.

Medium sized to larger defects can be treated by autologous chondrocyte implantation using the sandwich technology[2,8] (Fig.3).

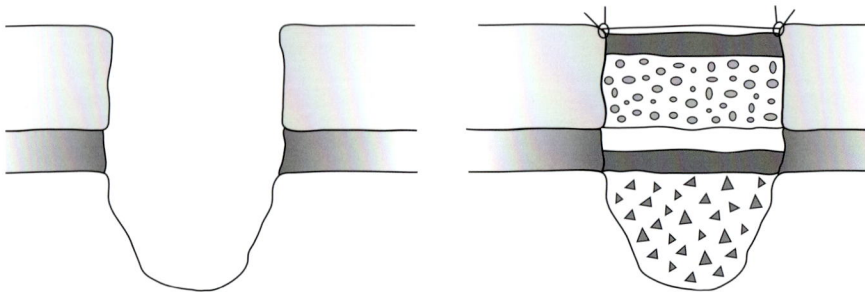

Figure 3: Medium sized to larger defects can be treated by autologous chondrocyte implantation using the sandwich technology; periosteum or collagen membranes cover the bone grafted area + periosteum or collagen membrane sutured over the cartilage defect. Cell suspension injected in between the two layers.

The bony defect is filled with bone grafts. Periosteum or a collagen membrane is put on top of the bone grafts in level with the subchondral bone plate and periosteum or a collagen membrane is sutured on top of the cartilage defect and the cells implanted in between the both membrane layers. The bone grafts used can be either autologous bone grafts, synthetic bone grafts or a combination of both. It is important to tightly pack the bone grafts by careful compression after a stimulation of the bone bottom to improve vascularization. The procedure can be done also transarthroscically with bone graft implanted via a tubular instrument followed by the type of cartilage graft used in combination with fibrin glue; bone paste + chondral graft[2] (Fig 4).

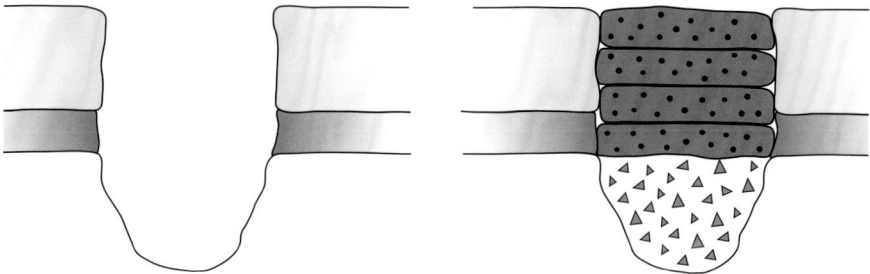

Figure 4: Transarthroscic osteochondral repair with bone graft implanted via a tubular instrument followed by the type of cartilage graft used in combination with fibrin glue; bone paste + chondral graft implanted in layers; "milles feuille technique".

Very large osteochondral defects are treated by osteochondral allografts[10]. An autologous alternative is the mega oats technology (Brucker et al. chapter 12).

Clinical data

Zazlav et al.[15] reported on a prospective clinical study to assess the effectiveness of autologous chondrocyte implantation in patients who failed prior treatments for articular cartilage defects of the knee. One hundred fifty-four patients with failed treatment for articular cartilage defects of the knee received autologous chondrocyte implantation in a multicenter, prospective study. Follow-up time was 48 months. Outcomes included change from baseline in knee function, knee pain, quality of life, and overall health. Duration of benefit after autologous chondrocyte implantation was compared with the failed prior cartilage repair procedure. One hundred twenty-six patients (82%) completed the protocol. Seventy-six percent of patients were treatment successes at study end, while 24% were regarded as treatment failures Mean improvements were observed from baseline to all time points (P < .001) for all outcome measures. Results did not differ between patients whose first surgery had been a marrow-stimulating procedure and those whose first procedure had been a debridement alone. The authors conclusion in that study was that patients with moderate to large chondral lesions with failed prior cartilage treatments can expect sustained and clinically meaningful improvement in pain and function after autologous chondrocyte implantation.

However, there are recent reports that marrow stimulation procedures may have a negative effect on subsequent repair of knee cartilage with autologous chondrocyte implantation, according to the results of a large cohort study.

In the Minas series of more than 300 patients who underwent autologous chondrocyte implantation (ACI), cartilage defects that were previously treated with marrow stimulation failed at three times the rate of defects that were not previously treated[12].

However, one may remember that most reports on ACI are on patients that had been treated before and those failed patients might have failed ACI also at first test. As for all comparisons, randomised studies are needed.

Conclusions

The patients need to know that cartilage surgery means three important things:

Time is long for the repair to mature into something that is biomechanically of functional quality.

Physiotherapy training postoperatively is extremely important for the patients to perform also for a long period.

Patience and tolerance is important for both the patient as well as the treating surgeon.

References

1. Brittberg M. Cell Carriers as the Next Generation of Cell Therapy for Cartilage Repair: A Review of the Matrix-Induced Autologous Chondrocyte Implantation Procedure. Am J Sports Med. 2009 Dec 4. (Epub ahead of print)

2. Brittberg M. Autologous chondrocyte implantation--technique and long-term follow-up. Injury. 2008 Apr;39 Suppl 1:S40-9

3. Brittberg M, Faxén E, Peterson L. Carbon fiber scaffolds in the treatment of early knee osteoarthritis. A prospective 4-year followup of 37 patients.Clin Orthop Relat Res. 1994 Oct;(307):155-64

4. Brittberg M, Winalski CS. Evaluation of cartilage injuries and repair. J Bone Joint Surg Am. 2003;85-A Suppl 2:58-69.

5. Carmont MR, Carey-Smith R, Saithna A, Dhillon M, Thompson P, Spalding T. Delayed incorporation of a TruFit plug: perseverance is recommended.Arthroscopy. 2009 Jul;25(7):810-4

6. Fulkerson J. Articular cartilage lesions in patellofemoral pain patients. In Disorders of the patellofemoral joint. Fulkerson JP, William and Wilkins, Baltimore 1997, 225-274.

7.Hangody L, Füles P. Autologous osteochondral mosaicplasty for the treatment of full-thickness defects of weight-bearing joints: ten years of experimental and clinical experience. J Bone Joint Surg Am. 2003;85-A Suppl 2:25-32

8.Jones DG, Peterson L. Autologous chondrocyte implantation.Instr Course Lect. 2007;56:429-45

9. Kon E, Delcogliano M, Filardo G, Fini M, Giavaresi G, Francioli S, Martin I, Pressato D, Arcangeli E, Quarto R, Sandri M, Marcacci M. Orderly osteochondral regeneration in a sheep model using a novel nano-composite multilayered biomaterial.J Orthop Res. 2009 Jul 21;28(1):116-124.

10.Lattermann C, Romine SE. Osteochondral allografts: state of the art. Clin Sports Med. 2009 Apr;28(2):285-301

11. Lu Y, Dhanaraj S, Wang Z, Bradley DM, Bowman SM, Cole BJ, Binette F. Minced cartilage without cell culture serves as an effective intraoperative cell source for cartilage repair. J Orthop Res. 2006

Jun;24(6):1261-70

12. Minas T, Gomoll AH, Rosenberger R, Royce RO, Bryant T. Increased failure rate of autologous chondrocyte implantation after previous treatment with marrow stimulation techniques. Am J Sports Med. 2009 May;37(5):902-8.

13. Pidoriano AJ, Weinstein RN, Buuck DA, Fulkerson JP. Correlation of patellar articular lesions with results from anteromedial tibial tubercle transfer.Am J Sports Med. 1997 Jul-Aug;25(4):533-7

14. Tognana E, Borrione A, De Luca C, Pavesio A. Hyalograft C: hyaluronan-based scaffolds in tissue-engineered cartilage.Cells Tissues Organs. 2007;186(2):97-103. Epub 2007 May 7. Review

15. Zaslav K, Cole B, Brewster R, DeBerardino T, Farr J, Fowler P, Nissen C; STAR Study Principal Investigators. .A prospective study of autologous chondrocyte implantation in patients with failed prior treatment for articular cartilage defect of the knee: results of the Study of the Treatment of Articular Repair (STAR) clinical trial.Am J Sports Med. 2009 Jan;37(1):42-55. Epub 2008 Oct 16.

"Drugs are not always necessary. Belief in recovery always is"

(Norman Cousins)

Chapter 19.

Rehabilitation Following Cartilage Injury and Repair Procedures

Dieter Van Assche, Barbara Wondrasch, May Arna Risberg

Take Home Message

- *Knowledge of the cartilage defect is of significance for the individualized rehabilitation program both for non-operatively treated and operatively treated articular cartilage injury*
- *Exercises and activities that modify joint loading is one of the key factors to reveal symptoms and improve function in patients with articular cartilage injuries*
- *Dynamic stability of the knee joint is of significance to generate sufficient amount of force in a timely fashion during exercises and activities*
- *Muscle strengthening exercises as well as neuromuscular exercises*

Introduction

Despite the fact that cartilage injuries have been recognized as a cause of significant morbidity for more then 200 years[2, 6] and that surgical techniques have been widely used for more than 15 years (ACI), the evidence for the effect of rehabilitation after cartilage injury or after surgery is more or less absent[17, 20]. But surgeons and physical therapists recognize that rehabilitation is of great significance to target impairments and disabilities reported in several studies in patients with articular cartilage injuries. Expert opinions, animal studies, basic science, applied biomechanics, published "current concepts", and clinical commentaries on

173

rehabilitation phases for patients with cartilage injuries, constitute the basis of knowledge for rehabilitation of patients with articular cartilage injuries or repair in the knee[3,6,8,12,14,17,19,21,36]. There is no evidence based guideline based on randomized controlled trials for rehabilitation after articular cartilage injuries or for postoperative rehabilitation programs after cartilage repair. The rehabilitation programs are based upon evidence from basic science, applied biomechanics, exercise physiology, clinical trials, and many years of clinical experience.

Randomized clinical trials on the effect of different rehabilitation programs are lacking. But some randomized controlled trials and long term outcome studies on the effect of *surgical procedures* such as marrow stimulation techniques, mosaicplasty, and ACI (autologous chondrocyte implantation) exist[18,24,34,43]. Furthermore, new technologies (e.g. better magnetic resonance imaging (MRI) techniques, including d'GEMRIC) have increased the knowledge on cartilage morphology and quality of articular cartilage in the knee at an early phase after injury and allow to assess changes in the articular cartilage over time, including after interventions[28,29,46,51,52].

Treatment strategies and rehabilitation guidelines depend upon the type and localization of the articular cartilage injury, the individualized patient's symptoms of pain and swelling, lower extremity function, the patient's activity level and goals, and the decision on articular cartilage repair or non-operative treatment. The overall aim is to reduce pain and swelling, and improve lower extremity function related to activities of daily living (ADL) and sport specific activities (the patient specific goals). The rehabilitation program could be either a preoperative rehabilitation program; optimizing the lower extremity function prior to surgery and preparing the individual for the upcoming surgical intervention and the postoperative rehabilitation, or it could be a non-operative treatment approach with the aim of returning the patient to his/her activity level. For patients going through surgical treatment, a preoperative rehabilitation program would be indicated and would be a significant intervention to achieve the best postoperative result.
Surgical treatment of articular cartilage injury with cell transplantation has shown to improve knee function[27,35] but has not shown to fully restore normal knee function in all patients[27,33]. Therefore, more evidence on significant predictors for developing normal knee function is required to enhance an improved outcome after articular cartilage injury, for injuries treated non-operatively or for those treated with cartilage repair.

The *main objective* of this chapter is to describe some of the current evidence within basic science, applied biomechanics, and clinical studies for rehabilitation after articular cartilage injury and repair. The aim is to describe current treatment approaches (rehabilitation phases) on relieving symptoms and improving lower extremity function for patients who go through a non-operative rehabilitation program or a preoperative rehabilitation program. Furthermore, to describe current treatment approaches for a rehabilitation program for those who go through articular cartilage repair.

Basic science and articular cartilage healing

Even though articular cartilage of human adults has no blood supply, chondrocytes show a high level of metabolism. Chondrocytes derive their nutrition mainly form synovial fluid and to a lesser extent form the underlying bone. They synthesise and assemble ECM (extracellular matrix) components and direct their distributions within the tissue. All this is in order to maintain the structure and function of the ECM. The high level of metabolism is mainly due to proteoglycans turnover[16,49]. For instance in the middle zone the half life of most proteoglycans is 2 to 3 months. Although collagen turnover takes place, its level is much lower. Hence, cartilage is capable of adapting to mechanical changes if chondrocytes are stimulated to increase matrix and collagen synthesis[23]. Acute trauma, overuse, or altered mechanics can contribute to cartilage breakdown by chondrocyte apoptosis (cell death) and decrease in proteoglycan synthesis, both resulting in loss of ECM[9,45]. Also changes in subchondral bone are known to enhance cartilage stress and breakdown. Repetitive or traumatic overload can create microfractures in the subchondral bone. Trabecular repair processes by callus formations and formation of new trabeculae can cause an increased stiffness of the subchondral region. This increased stiffness can result in decreased shock-absorbing properties of the subchondral region. Therefore this adaptive subchondral bone formation process may enhance increased cartilage stress and eventual cartilage degradation[50].

Articular cartilage healing is different since cartilage is avascular, aneural and alymphatic[7,26]. The repair process of vascularised tissue contains fibroblast or specific cells that must synthesize the repair tissue. Local cell proliferation or migration of cells from the wound area or from blood vessels entering the tissue, are responsible for local ECM production and repair tissue synthesis[44]. The absence of blood vessels and the very tight ECM, prohibit chondrocyte migration from adjacent healthy cartilage towards the wound. Both factors exclude a cell-based repair and cartilage regeneration[4]. So overall the natural healing capacity of articular cartilage is limited. Moreover, when articular cartilage injury occurs after the second decade of life, cartilage degradation occurs more rapidly. Ageing has been shown to change proliferation capacity, ECM production and responsiveness to growth factors stimulation[47]. In conclusion articular cartilage wound healing, when taking place, mostly is partial and most likely takes place in the younger subjects. The wound healing originates from proliferation of chondrocytes in the cartilage bordering the wound area.

The knowledge about the natural course of healing is limited; is the articular cartilage injury solely a focal injury or does it affect all the surrounding articular cartilage in the joint? A new MRI study has indicated that the whole articular cartilage seems to be affected by the injury[53]. This evidence, although yet limited, also needs to be considered for exercise therapy as well as for the surgical repair of the joint and postoperative rehabilitation programs.

Biomechanics and joint loading

Excessive joint forces have a potential to promote cartilage injuries by acute trauma, or through altered joint mechanics as a result of overuse injury. These changes in cartilage tissue may promote degenerative changes that in the long run may lead to development of osteoarthritis (OA). Cartilage injuries may occur as a result of an acute trauma or as a result of repetitive impulse loading of activities through the lifespan. Occurrence in adolescence or young adults may have potential consequences later in life. Repetitive impulse loading, such as running, delivers shock waves through the body across joint surfaces that could be harmful and expose the joints to degenerative changes over years[11,13].

During joint loading, normal articular cartilage acts as an important shock-transducer. Articular cartilage has approximately a total consolidation of 5% in vivo[11,13]. The amount of consolidation throughout the cartilage is highly non-uniform. The superficial zones of cartilage have different mechanical properties than the middle and deep layers. The superficial zone is characterized by high fluid flow (in and out), tensile surface strains and large compressive strains (> 50%). These compressive strains reduce to zero in the middle and deep regions of cartilage. The fluid exuded from the superficial layer in vivo gets trapped between the 2 articulating cartilage surfaces and maintains a high pressure level, thereby preventing the generation of high stresses and friction between the solid matrix elements of the articulating surfaces. In the middle and deep zones of articular cartilage there is a high concentration of proteoglycans content. Due to the negative charge of these proteogylcans, the ECM is hydrophilic and high amounts of water are attracted into the tissue, while the collagen network provides the tissue with tensile resistance to prevent unlimited expansion. The deeper layers are characterized by low fluid flow, fluid pressure and low compressive strains. These properties provide the middle and deep layers with stiffness against compression, needed for its role as a shock-transducer[5].

Besides these mechanical properties of articular cartilage an understanding of the applied clinical biomechanics must be considered. This is especially important when establishing rehabilitation guidelines including specific exercises for both non-operatively and operatively treated patients with articular cartilage injuries. Modifying joint loads is one of the key factors to relieve symptoms and improve function in patients with cartilage injuries. Many treatment approaches focus on either modifying joint loading or enhancement of the cartilage repair process. Treatment approaches for modifying joint loads include surgery, bracing and muscle strengthening exercises. All these interventions aim at changing the alignment to transfer load way from areas not tolerating high loads.
Animal experiments have provided considerable information about the effects of repetitive in vivo loading of articular cartilage[3,10]. It has been shown that loading with physiological mechanical forces is essential in maintaining normal state and function of articular cartilage and the subchondral bone[39,41]. Repetitive loading with physiologic mechanical forces even supports nutrition of the cartilage tissue by enhancing diffusion of synovial fluid[22,39,42].

On the contrary, studies have shown that unloading deteriorates the functional and structural properties of articular tissue by changing the biochemical composition[2,3,6,8]. These findings should be considered within the specific rehabilitation programs for patients with articular cartilage injuries.

The flexion and extension movement is a combination of rolling and gliding of the surface of the femur and the tibia linked up with a spin movement at the end of flexion and extension. To ensure a physiologic flexion and extension movement with a physiologic load distribution on the cartilage surfaces, restriction of these rolling and gliding as well as the spin movement should be avoided. The load distribution in the tibiofemoral joint should be considered in the choice and the progression of exercises.

The patellofemoral joint is a sellar joint composed of the patella and the underlying femoral trochlea. This joint is stabilized by active and passive stabilizers; active stabilizer is mainly the quadriceps muscle group and passive stabilizers are the femoral condyle, the peripatellar retinaculum, the medial and the lateral patellofemoral ligaments.

During flexion and extension the patella glides superiorly and inferiorly on the femur and only parts of the patella articulate with the femoral trochlea at any given time.

A smooth and unrestricted gliding of the patella on the trochlear groove help to distribute compression force over the whole patellofemoral joint and minimize joint reaction force. Cartilage lesions within this joint are often leading to reduced gliding of the patella which results in increased joint reaction forces and increased compression.

Beside these biomechanical findings, it is necessary to know the emerging loads during activities of daily life and during exercises.

Eckstein et al found a reduction in cartilage volume of the patella of 2.4 - 8.6% after 50 knee bends and he showed that after 100 knee bends there was no significant difference in the reduction of the cartilage volume[12]. Additionally he found a higher reduction of cartilage volume after static loading and periods of 90 minutes to attain the pre-exercise volume before the knee bends[12].

Comparing several activities such as knee bends, walking, running and cycling, running seems to cause the greatest amount of cartilage deformation whereas walking produces no massive reduction of cartilage volume[13]. Additionally it has been suggested that initial structural changes affect the subchondral bone especially when the joint is exposed to high impact loading[3].

These finding support the results of in-vitro investigations, however it only reveals the adaption and reaction of cartilage of healthy subjects. More research is necessary to evaluate the effects of exercise of injured cartilage tissue.

Muscle strength and neuromuscular control

The development of muscle strength and endurance is important to dissipate forces acting on the knee and in that way to protect the healing of the articular cartilage. Development of muscle strength and endurance is important to distribute forces acting on the knee and to protect the defect in the articular cartilage. The quadriceps muscle is often inhibited after injury and needs to be addressed in particular. Electrical stimulation and biofeedback are often applied to activate the quadriceps muscles, and several studies have examined the effect of electrical stimulation[15,25,36]. This quadriceps muscle is hence important as it acts as a shock absorber to the knee and helps to dissipate the ground reactions forces during weight bearing activities. Some authors recommend isometric exercises in the early phase as they produce no shear forces and minimize the risk for further damage. But this could be enhanced by electrical stimulation.

Muscle strengthening exercises aim at optimizing joint loading through improving alignment and improving the capabilities of the muscles as shock absorbers during activities. Today, there is a rationale why these exercises seem to relieve symptoms and improve function, and thereby a rationale for including them in the rehabilitation program. But more evidence and understanding on how these exercises work and especially the dose-response for normalizing knee function, are still lacking.

The understanding of contact forces, shear forces, and weight bearing areas of the knee during activities of daily living and sport activities are essential for the choice of exercises and the development and progression of exercises during the rehabilitation program.

Muscle force production can contribute to dynamic joint stability. The ability to generate sufficient amount of force in a timely fashion is of significance to maintain dynamic stability of the knee and limit excessive joint motion that may affect the static structures as ligaments and cartilage[19,31]. Muscle fatigue has shown to result in slower leg muscle responses and perturbation, and to increased anterior tibial translation, possibly resulting in decreased dynamic stability. Reaction to joint loading and how the knee joint copes with loading activities are also dependent on the neuromuscular function of the knee joint, in addition to the proximal and distal parts of the lower extremity, including the core stability. The core has also shown to have a significant impact on the loading of the lower extremity[1,55,56]. More recently insights in the quadriceps and the hip muscles (gluteus medius) functioning as shock absorbers during eccentric contractions may help to dissipate peak forces acting on the knee during weight-bearing activities. Muscle strengthening exercises as well as neuromuscular exercises are needed to change joint loading and improve lower extremity function.

The dynamic stability of the knee relies largely on proprioception, muscle strength, endurance, and power provided by the quadriceps, the hamstrings and the pelvis muscles during ADL and sport activities. So exercises that strengthen the entire lower extremity should be included in the later phases when strengthening exercises with relevant doses are tolerated. Core stability is also shown to be important to reduce load within the knee as good core stability assists in controlling the production and distribution of forces in the knee joint during activities. Further components of dynamic knee stabilization strategies are neuromuscular drills of the lower extremity (agility drills). Rehabilitation programs should therefore include exercises that improve the neuromuscular function such as using balance board exercises and other weight shifting activities, including pivoting activities, during the later return to sport phase.

Neuromuscular exercises are in addition to strengthening exercises the main types of exercises included in the rehabilitation programs for individuals with articular cartilage injuries. A few studies have also shown that including neuromuscular exercises prior to strength training exercises seems to improve muscle strength more than only including traditional strengthening exercises[37]. Neuromuscular exercises are also often better tolerated by the patients than only strengthening exercises.

I. Rehabilitation after articular cartilage injury in the knee

Successful non-operative treatment of articular cartilage lesions is based on patient's history, clinical examination, MRI, patient's goal, and not only local knee symptoms and function but the whole lower extremity function must be considered. The rehabilitation program for patients with articular cartilage injury could also be a preoperative rehabilitation program (Figure 1). Identifying the injury mechanism, local contributing factors of the knee, in addition to other affected parts of the lower extremity need to be included to target impairments and disabilities during the planned rehabilitation program[19,36,54].

Exercise therapy is prescribed to improve pain and function, but we do not know if the exercises in general (regarding both type and load) have a protective effect on joint structure or on cartilage in particular, neither do we know which exercises have a protective effect and which have a detrimental effect on joint structure. We lack knowledge on what joint loading is beneficial to the cartilage and in what stage of the healing process; also the time during the rehabilitation program the joint is susceptible to increased joint loading is still unknown. But long clinical experience, some clinical studies in addition to insight into the basic science and applied biomechanics form the basis for the outlined rehabilitation guidelines and rehabilitation phases stated below. These guidelines need to be included in future randomized controlled trials.

Pain and function are significant outcome parameters when examining the effect of exercise therapy. However, both the short term and long term effect on cartilage also need to be evaluated. Some studies have shown that exercises are efficient for decreasing pain and improving function but we have few studies that have reported long term consequences on the articular cartilage. However, we do know form several high quality randomized controlled trials that exercise therapy have shown to be effective in patients with knee OA. The changes in joint structure and the mechanisms for improved function are not clearly established. This highlights the importance of both basic science research on changes in joint loading and cartilage physiology in addition to clinical research for the short and long term effect of exercise therapy.

Type of lesions

Articular cartilage defects can be partial-thickness chondral defects, not necessarily associated with clinical problems, and they can be full-thickness chondral defects more commonly symptomatic with effusion and pain that affects lower extremity function and quality of life of individuals. These full-thickness cartilage defects (penetrating subchondral bone) have shown to have limited intrinsic repair capacity limited to production of hyaline cartilage tissue[7,26,32].

In young and active individuals the articular cartilage lesions are usually localized to 1 or 2 compartments of the knee joint and represent focal area that vary in size from small (<2cm²) to larger lesions (>8 cm²). These lesions can be present at the patella or trochlea, femur (medial or lateral condyle), or tibia. Insight into each of these lesion areas is needed to be able to include the right exercises, including the specific knee angle during exercises, and to understand the knee joint biomechanics during loading and during motion. Contact areas of the patellofemoral joint at different angles of knee flexion are essential for prescribing type of exercises for individuals with cartilage lesions of the patella. Similarly, understanding the biomechanics of the tibiofemoral joint during loading and at specific knee joint angles is essential for prescribing exercises for articular lesions of the femur or tibia. Furthermore, the size of the lesion and the location on the patella, femur, or tibia are also needed to understand why some exercises at specific knee angles are indicated and others not.

Individualization

Treatment modalities as well as rehabilitation have to address and treat the patients´ unique injuries and demands to support the return to desired activities.
The quality of articular cartilage is dependent upon several intrinsic factors including age, nutrition, body weight, joint alignment, type of injury, localization of injury, and extrinsic factors like work situation, sports activity level and previous injuries. All these factors are influencing rehabilitation and have therefore to be considered when designing and developing a rehabilitation program after cartilage injury.
The treatment plan of a patient with generalized osteoarthritis has to differ from the treatment plan of a young patient with a localized articular defect. Also the size and location of the lesion should influence the rehabilitation protocol by avoiding high shear forces over the defect size and stimulating the defect area in a physiologic and safe way. Therefore the applied clinical biomechanics have to be considered.

Pain and swelling are good indicators to assess and estimate the circulation situation of the joint and to get an idea about the status of joint homeostasis. Joint homeostasis can be described as a "quiet" and not inflamed condition of the joint, which is necessary for a joint and its structures to fulfil their functions.
The individual patient's pain and effusion are the two factors indicating if the

applied loads during the exercises or activities are optimal or not. Progression within the rehabilitation program should be performed in a manner that provides a healthy stimulus for the healing tissue.

Progression of load application

In the initial phase after injury all weight bearing activities should be controlled and limited. The dosage of exercises should be low and should be gradually increased with improvement of the patients' symptoms. For this reason the knowledge of the size and location of the lesion is important to appreciate the forces that will act on it. If the lesion is located in the weight bearing area of the femoral condyle, load should be limited by using crutches for at least three weeks. If the lesion is within the patellofemoral joint, ROM should be limited by using a brace. Weight bearing exercises and activities should be slowly increased and progression should be based on the symptoms of the patient.

Goal specific rehabilitation

The primary goal of rehabilitation after cartilage injury is to facilitate return to desired activities of the patient and to prevent the development of OA. Studies indicate that this can be achieved by enhanced lower extremity muscle strengthening and improved neuromuscular control. One of the main challenges during rehabilitation programs for patients with articular cartilage injury is to increase load and progression of exercises in a slow way, meaning without increased pain and swelling. Patient education should be included for optimal progression of exercises and adherence to the exercise protocol. The rehabilitation phases should be more criterion based than time based, and should be slowly progressed according to pain and swelling of the individual patients. Rehabilitation of patients with articular cartilage injuries requires more resources from the physical therapist compared to other knee injuries, due to the nature of the healing process that is much slower and because more time needs to be spent on patient education; progression of exercises and loading should be based on the patient's symptoms.

Treatment algorithm

Our clinical research group has established a treatment algorithm based on current evidence and recommendations.

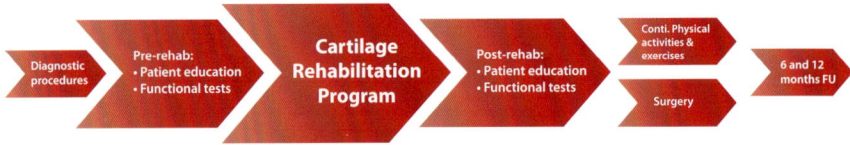

Figure 1: This figure shows the flow of patients with articular cartilage lesions. The patients first need to go through a specific diagnostic procedure including MRI, clinical examination, functional tests, prior to start of the individualized rehabilitation program. Post 3 months of rehabilitation the same clinical tests and functional tests are included before further treatment strategies are decided; either continuing exercise program or surgical interventions. 6 and 12 months following post rehabilitation or post surgery clinical and functional re-examinations are performed.

Phases	Therapeutic Aims	Milestones	Interventions / Exercises
Phase 1 'Protection' phase	Protection of the injured cartilage tissue against shearing and compression forces Decrease pain and swelling Normalize ROM Quadriceps control Normalize walking Patient education	- Full passive and active knee extension within 1 week - Flexion ROM only limited if related to type of lesions and location - Straight leg raising with active full knee extension - Quadriceps control during balance exercises - Quadriceps control during squatting - Symmetric weight bearing during exercises - Normal gait patterns with crutches	- Stationary bicycle – start with pendulum when knee flexion is <90°, advance to full cycle when knee flexion >90°, first without resistance - Isometric quadriceps contractions - Straight leg raising - Electrical quadriceps muscle stimulation - Manual patella mobilization - Squatting exercises with symmetric weight bearing, 10-60° of knee flexion - Balance exercises - Gait re-training - Cold therapy after exercise - Therapy

Phase 2 'Functional' phase	No or minimal swelling
	
	Normal gait patterns
	
	Normal two leg dynamic exercises
	
	Normal one leg dynamic exercises
	
	Two legs jump
	
	One leg jump
		- Normal gait on flat, even surface without crutches
		- Full active knee extension and hip control during one leg and two legs exercises
		- Stair climbing with hip and knee control
		- Walking for 30 minutes without pain or increased swelling
		- When no swelling, full ROM and active muscular control:
		  • Two leg jumping
		  • One leg jumping
		- Jogging on a treadmill
			- Stationary bicycle full ROM and with gradually increased resistance
			- Heel-raise exercises
			- Two leg squatting with symmetric weight bearing
			- Ascending and descending staircase exercises
			- Two leg balance exercises on uneven surface and BOSU balls
			- One leg squat on air inflated cushions
			- Leg curl - one leg
			- Hamstring exercises in slings and large gymnastic ball
			- Eccentric hamstring exercises
			- Dynamic stability exercises with increased speed
			- Bench press - one leg
			- Leg extension - one leg
			- Running on a treadmill
			- Two legs jumping exercises
			- One leg jumping exercises

| Phase 3 'Return to sports' phase | | - Prior to start Level 1 activities that include pivoting and jumping
- Isokinetic quadriceps muscle strength tests up to 15° knee extension1 > 90% compared to uninjured side. Maybe testing position should be different in defects within the PFJ and the TFJ? | - One leg squat on air inflated cushions with increased knee flexion
- Dynamic stability exercises with increased speed
- All strength exercises should include resistance exercise using the "+2 principles"2
  • Leg curl – one leg
  • Eccentric hamstring exercises
  • Bench press – one leg
  • Leg extension – one leg |

Table 1: Rehabilitation phases, therapeutic aims, milestones, and interventions. All aims, milestones and interventions are given within each phase with increased progression.

II. Rehabilitation of patients after cartilage repair procedures in the knee

Introduction: the evidence on rehabilitation after cell-based cartilage repair
Current scientific evidence on the impact of postoperative rehabilitation following knee cartilage repair is largely inadequate. For the autologous chondrocyte implantation (ACI) procedure, the evidence base for rehabilitation has been described as "in its infancy", which is a telling indictment[17]. While published reports of cartilage repair studies describe the surgical technique in great detail, the rehabilitation method and its possible effect on treatment efficacy are often overlooked. In fact, in a 2005 analysis of 61 cartilage repair studies, the description of postoperative rehabilitation in published reports was among the major methodology deficiencies highlighted by Jakobsen et al., who found only one study that mentioned compliance with rehabilitation[20]. This poses the question as to whether this gap in reporting is a simple oversight, or is it a sign of the lack of objective rehabilitation evidence?
Despite the fact that postoperative rehabilitation is clearly a treatment variable that will affect outcome, its role in the cartilage repair value chain and that of the physical therapist are for various reasons being underestimated (Figure 2).

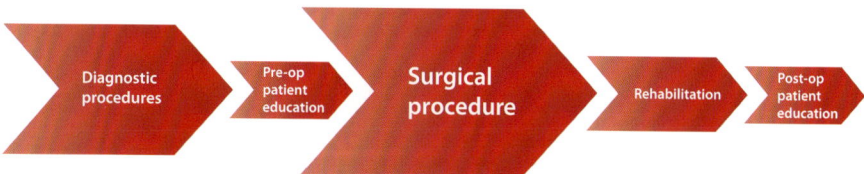

Figure 2: Cartilage repair value chain.

The true value of rehabilitation after cartilage injury or repair can be easily underestimated. Several basic factors could be identified, such as (1) the use of non-standardized protocols that are experience-based rather than evidence-based, (2) poor compliance with protocols, (3) lack of objective and or sensitive outcome measures, and (4) inadequate collaboration and communication. Therefore the main objective of this part II is to describe current evidence and recommendations for rehabilitation after cartilage repair.

A general guideline with aims and milestones

The most important conditions for complete recovery after cell based cartilage repair are created during the first 12 weeks of the rehabilitation process. Several groups have suggested general guidelines and they are all based upon the slow intrinsic biological process of cartilage formation, the protection of the repaired tissue post-surgery and an optimal functionality gain without jeopardizing the cartilage repair[14,17,54]. In table 2 a summary of rehabilitation phases is given, with the underlying biological process and general aims in rehabilitation. In addition a summary of therapeutic aims and milestones for progression are summarized in table 3. Therapeutic aims and milestone for progressing to a next phase are important. The time line is not to be taken strictly.

	Rehabilitation Phases	Biological Process and General Aims
1.	Preoperative phase	*Joint inflammation* Education on: 1/ rehabilitation planning 2/ Improve joint function 3/ prevention of excessive loads on affected zones Restoration of joint Homeostasis
2.	0-6 weeks post surgery	*Post-surgery joint inflammation and cell proliferation* Repair to complete ROM (range of motion) for defects < 5.0 cm^2 Achievement of homeostasis (no swelling or pain) in joint
3.	4-12 weeks post surgery	*Cell differentiation and start of maturation phase* Achievement of normal pattern of movement (muscle control) Improve specific strength within the safe zones
4.	10-26 weeks post surgery	*Cell differentiation, tissue formation, maturation phase* Maximizing physical fitness through low impact* activities (rowing and biking) or arm activities
5.	5-9 months post surgery	*Tissue formation and maturation* Increase muscle control within repaired zone Isometric control under high load in repaired zone Eccentric control: Full range during low impact High impact** within safe zones
6.	9-12 months post surgery	*Tissue formation and maturation* Sport-specific exercises for low impact sport allowed (no pivoting sports and open skills) High impact sports not allowed
7.	>12 months post surgery	*Maturation* Sport-specific exercises for high impact sports Low impact sport exercises

*Table 2: Rehabilitation phases in relation to rehabilitation aims based on classifications of Hambly et al, Gillogly et al, Reinhold et al. , *low impact: rowing and biking, ** high impact: pivoting sports, jogging, etc.*

Phases	Therapeutic Aims	Milestones

Phase 1.
Preoperative
phase
	– Education on:
	    • Rehabilitation planning
	    • Improve joint function
	    • Prevent excessive loads on affected
	      zones
	– Neuromuscular and proprioceptive training
	– Restoration of joint Homeostasis
		– Joint Homeostasis in rest
		– Informed patient
		– Surgical procedure for cartilage repair

Phase 2.
0-6 weeks
Post surgery
	– Protection of the healing tissue against shear
	  ing and compression forces (neuromuscular
	  and proprioceptive training)
	– Decrease of pain and swelling
	– Restoration of complete passive flexion
	– Gradual improvement of active flexion
	– Gain control over quadriceps and start general
	  physical fitness in no load conditions, f.i. using
	  upper limbs
		– Completion phase 2
		– Active flexion up to 110°
		– Minimal pain and swelling
		– If no swelling: complete passive flexion
		– Voluntary quadriceps activity in different knee
		  joint angles
		– Normal walking pattern at slow speed, with use
		  of 2 crutches

Phase 3.
4-12 weeks
Post surgery
	– Complete ROM as from 6 wks after surgery
	– Improve quadriceps strength and endurance
	– Improve functional activities and start general
	  physical fitness in low load conditions
	– Extend load according to defined aims
	– Maintain homeostasis (pain, swelling)
	– Aim for a good walking pattern and prevent
	  'anterior knee pain' (from reduced active
	  stability) by neuromuscular training
		– Completion of phase 3
		– Minimal pain and swelling
		– Full active ROM
		– No reactive knee (increase of pain and swelling)
		  after strength exercises
		– Able to walk 1.6 – 3.2 km or bike and/or row 30
		  minutes on an ergometer

Phase 4.
10–26 weeks
Post surgery
	– Improve muscle strength within safety margin
	– Improve specific muscle endurance through
	  'low impact' activities or exercises
	– Extend functional activities
	– Maximize general physical fitness in low load
	  conditions
		– Completion of phase 4
		– No pain or swelling during 'low impact'
		  exercises
		– Full active, painless ROM
		– Strength within 75-80% of contralateral leg
		– Balance and stability within 75 - 80% of
		  contralateral leg

Phase 5.
5-9 months
Post surgery
	– Muscle control within loaded zone
	– Extend functional activities
	– The strength and functionality evaluation if
	  patient experiences no pain or swelling.
	– Improve physical fitness exercises also using
	  moderate load conditions
		– Completion of phase 5
		– No pain or swelling during or after 'low impact'
		  or 'high impact' exercises

Phase 6.
9-12 months
Post surgery
	– Sport-specific training, 'low impact' sports
	– The strength and functionality evaluations are
	  advisable to adapt setting of goals
	– Improve physical fitness exercises using
	  moderate load conditions
		– Completion of phase 6
		– No pain or swelling during or after long
		  intervals of 'low impact' sports or 'high impact'
		  exercises with short time intervals
		– Strength within 85% of non-operated leg
		– Balance and stability within 85% of non-
		  operated leg

Phase 7.
>12 months
post surgery
	– Maximize sport- or work-specific training to
	  'high impact' activities.
	– Unrestricted return to 'low impact' sports
	– The strength and functionality evaluation if
	  patient needs to progress further and/or goals
	  setting needs adaptation
		– Completion of phase 7
		– No pain or swelling during or after 'high impact'
		  training sessions
		– Full recovery of sport specific strength
		  endurance
		– Strength within 90% of non-operated leg
		– Balance and stability within 90% of
		  non-operated leg

Table 3: Rehabilitation phases following cartilage repair, therapeutic aims and milestones.

General principles and modalities

Nutrition and joint circulation exercises

Chondrocytes derive their nutrition mainly from synovial fluid. Synovial fluid has a high viscosity under static joint compression and during rest (no joint motion). From the start joint motion takes place, minor shear forces act on the synovial fluid. Consequently the viscosity drops locally and the synovial fluid is temporarily 'water-like'. In this 'water-like' state the diffusion is facilitated through the cartilage and chondrocyte nutrition is promoted[57]. Joint circulation exercises are exercises with the accent on improving the general joint metabolism. The synovial fluid production is stimulated and the diffusion between synovial fluid and cartilage facilitated. So it's preferable that joint circulation exercises are in low-load conditions and over a wide range of motion. Continuous passive motion (CPM) is the most well-known joint circulation modality. Besides the effect of preventing joint arthrofibrosis post-surgery, several animal studies and a few studies in humans show a significant benefit of CPM compared to immobilization[40]. The optimal dose of joint circulation exercises is un-known. Often the use of CPM is promoted 6 to 8 hours a day[38]. Overall it is believed that these exercises play an essential role since nourishment and stimulation of the transplanted cells can be done early, effective and safe. If the cells receive daily nourishment, they can properly develop and become optimally integrated in their surroundings. To summarize the joint circulation exercises must be: repetitive with a large ROM, painless, performed daily and for a longer period of time, for example 15 minutes or more, several times a day, easy to perform, safe and preferably active and without substantial load.

Joint circulation exercises are necessary during each rehabilitation phase; without nourishment, cell and tissue adaptations are not possible. Several modalities are possible, such as CPM, Heel slides, Cycling and Rowing. Cycling and Rowing are possible without resistance and preferred with the feet attached. Rowing is an attractive alternative for cycling in the post-surgical training since the range of motion can be controlled well and the movement control is easier compared to cycling. On the bike often only the push phase is controlled well by the opposite leg and consequently the operated leg is passively flexed in uncontrolled manner[17].

Protection and injury prevention post-surgery

Several rehabilitation protocols point out the use of bracing the first 6 to 8 weeks after cartilage surgery. Depending on the indication we can distinguish two types of bracing: the post-operative brace and the 'functional unloader' brace. The post-operative brace helps the patient to restrict specific movement ranges and provides comfort to rest. The brace is a double-hinge type with flexion and extension range controlled at the axis of the hinges. Following patello-femoral cartilage repair, for example, the patient is allowed to weight bear directly in full extension. Restricting the flexion mobility during gait is sensible because when the knee would be loaded in flexed position the chance of delamination or damaging the graft is high. A simple sit to stand maneuver in the week post surgery without protection could be harmful. A post-operative brace is helpful to gradually allow range of motion and maximize participation in activities of daily living in safe conditions.

In contrast to patello-femoral repair, the tibio-femoral cartilage repair is less vulnerable to shear load by range of motion issues. Tibio-femoral cartilage repair can be easily overloaded when resuming gait or functional loading from sit to stand, doing stairs, etc… If it is accompanied by mal-alignment or insufficient postural control the peak load will even be greater. Since both factors are often present in patients with cartilage repair the type of 'functional unloader' brace is often prescribed for the months following cartilage repair. The functional unloader can be double- or single-hinge type. The hinge is poly-axial to mimic normal arthrokinematica of the knee movement[30]. The 'unloader brace' pushes the knee slightly to varus or valgus alignment for respectively repairs in the lateral and medial compartment of the knee. In this manner the peak load is avoided during lengthy functional activities. In patients with medial knee osteoarthritis these braces show efficient reduction in pain and functional disabilities. To summarize: the 'unloader brace' is often suggested for patients with mal-alignment and or proximal insufficient muscle control. With the use of an 'unloader brace' the peak loads can be controlled over the repair site and the patient can exercise for the gain in functionality.

To prevent re-injury the cause of the first trauma needs to be elucidated. Quite often several factors, intrinsic and extrinsic, can be identified contributing to the susceptibility to cartilage injury. Educating the possible risk factors to re-injury and the need to exercise to overcome the risks is more than necessary. Appropriate training schedule, shoes, sport level, sleep, intensity, load, underground, motivation, proximal muscle control, etc… can play an important role in getting the preset goal or not.

Furthermore systematic evaluation of goals and functionality is a necessity for an individualized rehabilitation. Since functional gains and tissue adaptations are generally slow after cartilage repair we suggest evaluations of for instance strength and hop function at 6, 9, 12 and 24 months after surgery.

From a general guideline to an individual rehabilitation program

Before surgery and at different stages in rehabilitation after surgery it is important to educate / coach / guide the patient to optimize functionality. The use of a visual overview with different accents of rehabilitation is very helpful. (Figure 3).

Overview rehabilitation goals and accents

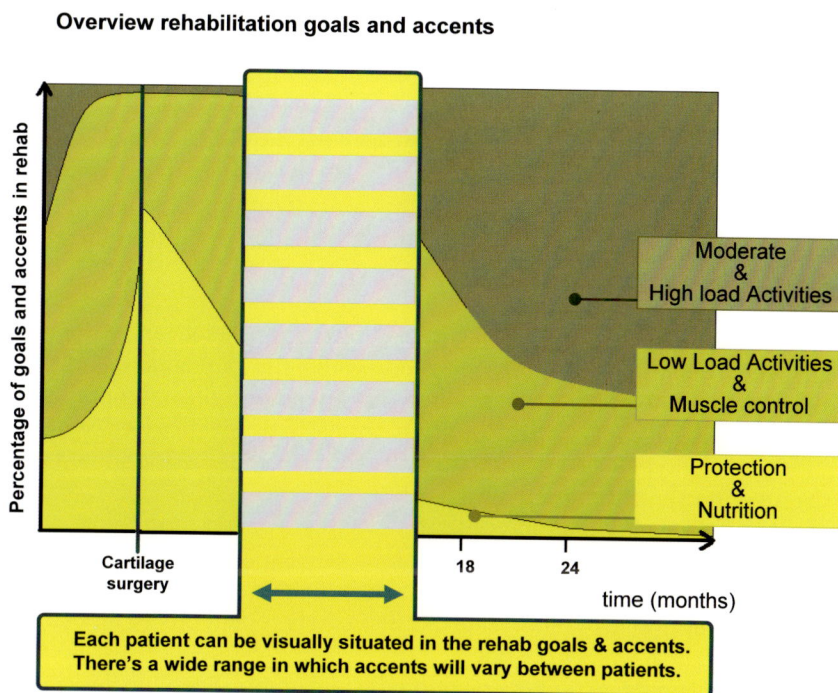

Figure 3: *Overview of rehabilitation goals and and accents.*

The general guidelines for rehabilitation must be individualized, since each patient is unique and recovers differently. So rehabilitation is without a doubt very individual. Beside personal factors, such as age, motivation, social support, the following factors are interesting to take into account as physical therapist:
1. Exact location of the repair (superior, middle, inferior or anterior, middle, posterior)
2. Size of the repair (<2,5cm²>)
3. Condition of the borders of the repair, (contained or not contained)
4. Duration of symptoms before surgery (<12 months>)
5. Pre-injury activity level (professional/non-professional, competitive/non-competitive, high/low knee impact and high/low training volume)
6. Movement dysfunctions in lower extremity or core
7. Changes in body mass index

There's evidence that these factors influence functional outcome in patients with cartilage disorders or in patients with cell based cartilage repair.

An individual approach based upon repair characteristics on the femur condyle

In table 4 an overview is given on how to adapt training post-surgery in order to avoid excessive shear stress and to improve the resistance to strain of the re-paired tissue by controlled loading for the tibio-femoral joint. Three factors of the repair site were taken into account: the exact location of the repair, the size of the repair ($<2,5cm^2>$) and the condition of the borders of the repair (contained or not contained).

Controlling shear stress and loading in the tibio-femoral joint can be done by:
— Avoiding weight on the leg when moving within the joint angles mentioned. Practical: the use of 2 crutches is advised as long as the aims of continued joint homeostasis are not achieved. It is normal to experience local swelling and pain during the first month after surgery. Pain and swelling should not occur during and after exercises.
— Avoiding slow or long-lasting positions over the repaired zone before or during training.
— When training over the repaired zone aim to do it on an intermittent base. For instance perform many short sets of 5 movement repetitions 10 times, rest of 20 seconds, 3 to 5 times per day.
— Learn to change directions by pivoting the feet in semi knee/hip flexion and control leg rotations by improvement of hip muscle control.
— Use objective feedback of weight bearing within joint angels mentioned during Closed Kinetic Chain (CKC) exercises. To assess the load you can use a simple weight scale. It is much easier to control the amount of weight bearing in static positions compared to dynamic movement such as squatting. There-fore aim on using the weight scales during the dynamic exercises, with and without feedback on the weight.
— Slowly progress intensity of load within a high training volume at normal movement speeds.
— Always exercise with an optimal proximal muscle control, do not allow any movement dysfunctions.

Location on femur	Repair size (cm²) and borders	Avoid shear-stress between	Intermittent controlled loading in CKC between
Anterior	< 2.5	0° to 30° flexion	0° to 40° flexion
	> 2.5, contained	0° to 60° flexion	0° to 70° flexion
	> 2.5, uncontained	0° to 110° flexion	0° to 120° flexion
Central	< 2.5	20° - 80° flexion	10° - 90° flexion
	> 2.5, contained	20° - 110° flexion	10° - 120° flexion
	> 2.5, uncontained	10° - 120° flexion	0° - 130° flexion
Posterior	< 2.5	45° - 130° flexion	35° - 140° flexion
	> 2.5, contained	45° - 130° flexion	35° - 140° flexion
	> 2.5, uncontained	45° – full flexion	35° – full flexion

Table 4: An overview of training suggestions for a repair on the femoral condyle taking location, size and border into account.

An individual approach based upon repair characteristics in the patella-femoral joint

In table 5 an overview is given in on how to adapt training post-surgery in order to avoid excessive shear stress and to improve the resistance to strain of the repaired tissue by controlled loading for the patella-femoral joint.

Controlling shear stress and load in the patella-femoral joint is more complex:

– Overall the first 3 to 5 months open kinetic chain exercises over the repair zone to strengthen the quadriceps need to be avoided. The excessive stress during repetitive open kinetic chain movement easily damages repair tissue. Open kinetic chain exercises can be done in ranges not stressing the repair tissue. Use above mentioned CKC exercises. The load on the patella will increase a lot during fast eccentric muscle work of the Quadriceps. So when training on eccentric movement control, such as during leg press on one leg, try to decrease the power output first. Take low resistance and improve muscle control of the full range. Before increasing weight adapt the movement speed.

The faster the movement speed the higher the load. Since the cause of patella lesions is often instability, the accent on neuromuscular control is essential. Objective feedback on weight bearing is for the patella-femoral joint load only one of several influencing factors. Therefore aim on controlling movement speed, movement direction, proximal muscle control and the weight or load pushed away or better controlled during a landing maneuver.

− When training over the repaired zone aim to control the direction of movement within the closed chain exercise. For instance when pushing the positioned foot forward to the knee position during a backward push off, the concentric quadriceps function will stress much more the patella-femoral joint compared to a forward push of or a forward lunge. During forward lunge the strength will be generated more by the hip extensors.

− When training over the repaired zone aim to do it on an intermittent base. For instance perform short sets (5 movement repetitions) many times (10), rest in between 10 seconds, 3 to 5 times per day.

− Avoid slow or long-lasting positions with stress on the repaired zone at rest, before or during training.

− Slowly progress intensity of load over the repair zone within a high training volume at normal movement speeds.

− Always exercise with an optimal proximal muscle control, do not allow any movement dysfunctions.

Location on		Repair size (cm²) and borders	Avoid shear-stress between	Intermittent controlled loading in CKC between
Patella	Trochlea			
Inferior	*Superior*	< 2.5	0° to 30° flexion	0° to 30° flexion
		> 2.5, contained	0° to 40° flexion	0° to 40° flexion
		> 2.5, uncontained	0° to 40° flexion	0° to 60° flexion
Central	*Central*	< 2.5	20° - 75° flexion	20° - 75° flexion
		> 2.5, contained	10° - 85° flexion	10° - 85° flexion
		> 2.5, uncontained	10° - 85° flexion	5° - 90° flexion
Superior	*Inferior*	< 2.5	45° - 130° flexion	35° - 140° flexion
		> 2.5, contained	45° - 130° flexion	35° - 140° flexion
		> 2.5, uncontained	45° – full flexion	35° – full flexion

Table 5: An overview of training suggestions for a repair in the patellofemoral joint, taking location, size and border into account.

References

1. Abt J; Smoliga J; Brick M; Jolly J; Lephart S; Fu F, Relationship between cycling mechanics and core stability, J Strength.Cond.Res, 2007, 21:1300-1304.
2. Alford J; Cole B, Cartilage restoration, part 1: basic science, historical perspective, patient evaluation, and treatment options, Am.J.Sports Med, 2005,33:295-306.
3. Arokoski J; Jurvelin J; Vaatainen U; Helminen H, Normal and pathological adaptations of articular cartilage to joint loading, Scand.J.Med.Sci.Sports, 2000,10:186-198.
4. Bos P; Kops N; Verhaar J; van Osch G, Cellular origin of neocartilage formed at wound edges of articular cartilage in a tissue culture experiment, Osteoarthritis.Cartilage, 2008,16:204-211.
5. Boschetti F; Peretti G, Tensile and compressive properties of healthy and osteoarthritic human articular cartilage, Biorheology, 2008, 45:337-344.
6. Buckwalter J, Effects of early motion on healing of musculoskeletal tissues, Hand Clin, 1996,12:13-24.
7. Buckwalter J; Mankin H; Grodzinsky A, Articular cartilage and osteoarthritis, Instr.Course Lect, 2005, 54:465-480.
8. Buschmann M; Gluzband Y; Grodzinsky A; Hunziker E, Mechanical compression modulates matrix biosynthesis in chondrocyte/agarose culture, J Cell Sci, 1995, 108 (4):1497-1508.
9. Carter D; Beaupre G; Wong M; Smith R; Andriacchi T; Schurman D; Smith R, The mechanobiology of articular cartilage development and degeneration, Clin.Orthop, 2004, S69-S77.
10. Cohen N; Foster R; Mow V, Composition and dynamics of articular cartilage: structure, function, and maintaining healthy state, J Orthop Sports Phys Ther, 1998, 28:203-215.
11. Eckstein F; Faber S; Muhlbauer R; Hohe J; Englmeier K; Reiser M; Putz R, Functional adaptation of human joints to mechanical stimuli, Osteoarthritis.Cartilage, 2002, 10:44-50.
12. Eckstein F; Hudelmaier M; Putz R, The effects of exercise on human articular cartilage. J.Anat, 2006, 208:491-512.
13. Eckstein F; Lemberger B; Gratzke C; Hudelmaier M; Glaser C; Englmeier K; Reiser M, In vivo cartilage deformation after different types of activity and its dependence on physical training status, Ann. Rheum.Dis, 2005, 64:291-295.
14. Gillogly S; Myers T; Reinold M, Treatment of full-thickness chondral defects in the knee with autologous chondrocyte implantation, J Orthop Sports Phys Ther, 2006, 36:751-764.
15. Goodwin P; Morrissey M, Physical therapy after arthroscopic partial meniscectomy: is it effective? Exerc.Sport Sci.Rev, 2003, 31:85-90.
16. Haapala J; Lammi M; Inkinen R; Parkkinen J; Agren U; Arokoski J; Kiviranta I; Helminen H; Tammi M, Coordinated regulation of hyaluronan and aggrecan content in the articular cartilage of immobilized and exercised dogs, J.Rheumatol, 1996, 23:1586-1593.
17. Hambly K; Bobic V; Wondrasch B; Van Assche D; Marlovits S, Autologous chondrocyte implantation postoperative care and rehabilitation: science and practice, Am.J.Sports Med, 2006, 34:1020-1038.
18. Hangody L; Vasarhelyi G; Hangody L; Sukosd Z; Tibay G; Bartha L; Bodo G, Autologous osteochondral grafting--technique and long-term results, Injury, 2008, 39 Suppl 1:S32-S39.
19. Irrgang J; Pezzullo D, Rehabilitation following surgical procedures to address articular cartilage lesions in the knee, J.Orthop.Sports Phys.Ther, 1998, 28:232-240.
20. Jakobsen R; Engebretsen L; Slauterbeck J, An analysis of the quality of cartilage repair studies, J.Bone Joint Surg.Am, 2005, 87:2232-2239.
21. Jurvelin J; Kiviranta I; Tammi M; Helminen H, Effect of physical exercise on indentation stiffness of articular cartilage in the canine knee, Int.J.Sports Med, 1986, 7:106-110.
22. Kiviranta I; Tammi M; Jurvelin J; Saamanen A; Helminen H, Moderate running exercise augments glycosaminoglycans and thickness of articular cartilage in the knee joint of young beagle dogs, J.Orthop.Res, 1988, 6:188-195.
23. Knecht S; Vanwanseele B; Stussi E, A review on the mechanical quality of articular cartilage - implications for the diagnosis of osteoarthritis, Clin.Biomech, 2006, 21:999-1012.
24. Kon E; Verdonk P; Condello V; Delcogliano M; Dhollander A; Filardo G; Pignotti E; Marcacci M, Matrix-Assisted Autologous Chondrocyte Transplantation for the Repair of Cartilage Defects of the Knee: Systematic Clinical Data Review and Study Quality Analysis, Am.J Sports Med, 2009, 37:S156-S66.
25. Lin F; Wilson N; Makhsous M; Press J; Koh J; Nuber G; Zhang L, In vivo patellar tracking induced by individual quadriceps components in individuals with patellofemoral pain, J Biomech, 2009, 43:235-41.
26. Mankin H, The response of articular cartilage to mechanical injury, J Bone Joint Surg.Am, 1982,

64:460-466.

27. Marcacci M; Berruto M; Brocchetta D; Delcogliano A; Ghinelli D; Gobbi A; Kon E; Pederzini L; Rosa D; Sacchetti GL; Stefani G; Zanasi S, Articular cartilage engineering with Hyalograft C: 3-year clinical results, Clin.Orthop Relat Res, 2005, 96-105.

28. Marlovits S; Singer P; Zeller P; Mandl I; Haller J; Trattnig S, Magnetic resonance observation of cartilage repair tissue (MOCART) for the evaluation of autologous chondrocyte transplantation: Determination of interobserver variability and correlation to clinical outcome after 2 years, Eur.J.Radiol, 2006, 57:24-31.

29. Marlovits S; Striessnig G; Resinger C; Aldrian S; Vecsei V; Imhof H; Trattnig S, Definition of pertinent parameters for the evaluation of articular cartilage repair tissue with high-resolution magnetic resonance imaging, Eur.J.Radiol, 2004, 52:310-319.

30. Matsuno H; Kadowaki K; Tsuji H, Generation II knee bracing for severe medial compartment osteoarthritis of the knee, Arch.Phys Med.Rehabil, 1997, 78:745-749.

31. McGinty G; Irrgang J; Pezzullo D, Biomechanical considerations for rehabilitation of the knee, Clin. Biomech, 2000, 15:160-166.

32. Nakamae A; Engebretsen L; Bahr R; Krosshaug T; Ochi M, Natural history of bone bruises after acute knee injury: clinical outcome and histopathological findings, Knee.Surg.Sports Traumatol. Arthrosc, 2006, 14:1252-8.

33. Nehrer S; Domayer S; Dorotka R; Schatz K; Bindreiter U; Kotz R, Three-year clinical outcome after chondrocyte transplantation using a hyaluronan matrix for cartilage repair. Eur.J.Radiol. 2006, 57:3-8.

34. Nehrer S; Dorotka R; Domayer S; Stelzeneder D; Kotz R, Treatment of Full-Thickness Chondral Defects With Hyalograft C in the Knee: A Prospective Clinical Case Series With 2 to 7 Years' Follow-up, Am.J Sports Med, 2009, 37:S81-S87.

35. Peterson L; Minas T; Brittberg M; Nilsson A; Sjogren-Jansson E; Lindahl A, Two- to 9-year outcome after autologous chondrocyte transplantation of the knee, Clin.Orthop, 2000, 212-234.

36. Reinold M; Wilk K; Macrina L; Dugas J; Cain E, Current concepts in the rehabilitation following articular cartilage repair procedures in the knee, J Orthop Sports Phys Ther, 2006, 36:774-794.

37. Risberg M; Holm I; Myklebust G; Engebretsen L, Neuromuscular training versus strength training during first 6 months after anterior cruciate ligament reconstruction: a randomized clinical trial, Phys Ther, 2007, 87:737-750.

38. Rodrigo J, Improvement of full-thickness chondral defect healing in the human knee after debridement and microfracture using CPM, Am.J.Knee Surg, 1994, 7:109-116.

39. Sah R; Kim Y; Doong J; Grodzinsky A; Plaas A; Sandy J, Biosynthetic response of cartilage explants to dynamic compression, J Orthop Res, 1989, 7:619-636.

40. Salter R, The biologic concept of continuous passive motion of synovial joints; The first 18 years of basic research and its clinical application, Clin.Orthop.Relat Res, 1989, 12-25.

41. Salter R, The physiologic basis of continuous passive motion for articular cartilage healing and regeneration, Hand Clin, 1994, 10:211-219.

42. Salter R; Simmonds D; Malcolm B; Rumble E; MacMichael D; Clements N, The biological effect of continuous passive motion on the healing of full-thickness defects in articular cartilage; An experimental investigation in the rabbit; J Bone Joint Surg.Am, 1980, 62:1232-1251.

43. Saris D; Vanlauwe J; Victor J; Almqvist K; Verdonk R; Bellemans J; Luyten F, Treatment of Symptomatic Cartilage Defects of the Knee: Characterized Chondrocyte Implantation Results in Better Clinical Outcome at 36 Months in a Randomized Trial Compared to Microfracture, Am.J Sports Med, 2009, 37:S10-119.

44. Shapiro F; Koide S; Glimcher M, Cell origin and differentiation in the repair of full-thickness defects of articular cartilage, J Bone Joint Surg.Am, 1993, 75:532-553.

45. Smith R; Carter D; Schurman R, Pressure and shear differentially alter human articular chondrocyte metabolism: a review, Clin.Orthop, 2004, S89-S95.

46. Trattnig S; Mamisch T; Pinker K; Domayer S; Szomolanyi P; Marlovits S; Kutscha-Lissberg F; Welsch G, Differentiating normal hyaline cartilage from post-surgical repair tissue using fast gradient echo imaging in delayed gadolinium-enhanced MRI (dGEMRIC) at 3 Tesla, Eur.Radiol, 2008, 18:1251-9.

47. van Osch G; Brittberg M; Dennis J; Bastiaansen-Jenniskens Y; Erben R; Konttinen Y; Luyten F, Cartilage repair: past and future, J Cell Mol.Med, 2009, 13:792-810.

48. Van Wingerden B (ed), Connective Tissue in Rehabilitation, Vaduz, Liechtenstein, Scipro Verlag, 1995.

49. Vanwanseele B; Lucchinetti E; Stussi E, The effects of immobilization on the characteristics of articular cartilage: current concepts and future directions, Osteoarthritis &Cartilage, 2002, 10:408-419.

50. vies-Tuck M; Wluka A; Wang Y; Teichtahl A; Jones G; Ding C; Cicuttini F, The natural history of cartilage defects in people with knee osteoarthritis, Osteoarthritis.Cartilage, 2008, 16:337-342.

51. Welsch G; Mamisch T; Domayer S; Dorotka R; Kutscha-Lissberg F; Marlovits S; White LM; Trattnig S, Cartilage T2 assessment at 3-T MR imaging: in vivo differentiation of normal hyaline cartilage from reparative tissue after two cartilage repair procedures--initial experience, Radiology, 2008, 247:154-161.

52. Welsch G; Mamisch T; Marlovits S; Glaser C; Friedrich K; Hennig F; Salomonowitz E; Trattnig S, Quantitative T2 mapping during follow-up after matrix-associated autologous chondrocyte transplantation (MACT): full-thickness and zonal evaluation to visualize the maturation of cartilage repair tissue, J Orthop Res, 2009, 27:957-963.

53. Welsch G; Mamisch T; Weber M; Horger W; Bohndorf K; Trattnig S, High-resolution morphological and biochemical imaging of articular cartilage of the ankle joint at 3.0 T using a new dedicated phased array coil: in vivo reproducibility study, Skeletal Radiol, 2008, 37:519-526.

54. Wilk K; Briem K; Reinold M; Devine K; Dugas J; Andrews J, Rehabilitation of articular lesions in the athlete's knee, J Orthop Sports Phys Ther, 2006, 36:815-827.

55. Zazulak B; Hewett T; Reeves N; Goldberg B; Cholewicki J, Deficits in neuromuscular control of the trunk predict knee injury risk: a prospective biomechanical-epidemiologic study, Am.J Sports Med, 2007, 35:1123-1130.

56. Zazulak B; Hewett T; Reeves N; Goldberg B; Cholewicki J, The effects of core proprioception on knee injury: a prospective biomechanical-epidemiological study, Am.J Sports Med, 2007, 35:368-373.

57. Zhang L; Gardiner B; Smith D; Pivonka P; Grodzinsky A, The effect of cyclic deformation and solute binding on solute transport in cartilage, Arch.Biochem.Biophys, 2007, 457:47-56.

"The Voyage of discovery lies not in seeking new horizons, but in seeing with new eyes "

(Marcel Proust)

Chapter 20.

Future of Cartilage Treatment

Alberto Gobbi , Henning Madry, Giuseppe Peretti

Take Home Message

For successful future cartilage tissue engineering a solid collaboration of experts from different disciplines, like chemistry, physics, biology, engineering, imaging, medicine and surgery are needed. This possibly would lead to the generation of tissue engineered strategies for the repair of complex lesions involving cartilage, together with the subchondral bone.
To be improved is the degree of bonding and integration of newly formed tissue as well as to find the most suitable chondrogenic and osteogenic cells for a perfect repair.

Introduction

As early as 1743, Hunter recognized that "articular cartilage lesions don't heal"; the limited intrinsic healing potential of articular cartilage is attributed to the presence of few and specialized cells with a low mitotic activity[1]. Another property of articular cartilage that limits its reparative ability is due to the fact that cartilage is avascular. Therefore, once injury occurs, surgical intervention may be necessary to achieve repair of the resulting focal chondral defects to obtain good functional outcome.

Nonsurgical treatment of cartilage lesions, including diet, intra-articular injections, and rehabilitation were relegated to pain control and activity modifications. However, recent studies on pulsed electromagnetic fields[2] have shown that these methods have the capacity to help heal cartilage tissue and delay osteoarthritis.

Massari et al.[3] summarized the results of the translational research of the Cartilage Repair and Electromagnetic Stimulation study group on the use of specific pulsed electromagnetic fields (I-ONE; IGEA, Carpi, Italy) (Figure 1) to control local joint inflammation and, ultimately, to have a chondroprotection effect on articular cartilage.

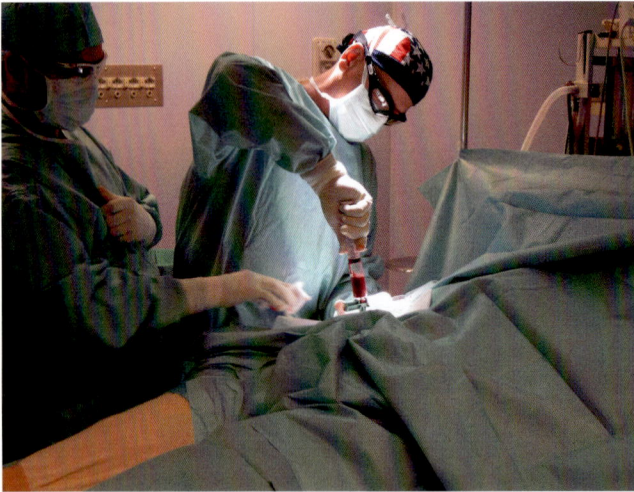

Figure 1: Bone marrow aspiration.

The study showed that of patients who underwent chondral coblation at 3-year follow-up, the number of patients who completely recovered was higher in the group treated with I-ONE therapy compared with the control group. Clinical results show how I-ONE therapy is an effective chondroprotective treatment for patients immediately after arthroscopic surgery without any negative side effects and exerts a short-term effect in reducing functional recovery time.

Traditional surgical techniques that are palliative (i.e. lavage, chondroplasty) only provide symptomatic pain relief with no actual hyaline tissue formation. Bone marrow stimulation techniques (i.e. microfracture, drilling) produce fibrocartilaginous tissue that will degenerate with time. Autologous osteochondral grafts and mosaicplasty restore normal cartilage tissue, but the application is restricted to small defects and there are some concerns about donor-site morbidity.

First generation autologous chondrocyte implantation (ACI), introduced by Peterson has been proven capable of restoring hyaline cartilage tissue[4]. Recent studies suggested the durability of this treatment, especially at long-term follow up, primarily due to its ability to produce hyaline-like cartilage that is mechanically and functionally stable even in athletes, however, this method requires 2 surgical procedures and showed local morbidity for periosteal harvest[5].

Second generation ACI represents a modern and viable technique for cartilage full thickness chondral lesion repair[6,7]. Aside from the risk of harvest site morbidity and two surgical procedures, the total cost of the operation, scaffold and process of chondrocyte cell culture is still very high.

At present the most promising technique seems to be ortho biolologics and one step surgery. Mesenchymal stem cells (MSC), platelet rich plasma (PRP) and tissue engineering, where cells are combined with scaffolds to pre-form a given tissue could be a new solution to cartilage repair.

Mesenchymal Stem Cell

Recent directions in cartilage repair are moving towards the possibility to perform one-step surgery: these could include the use of mesenchymal stem cells (MSC) and growth factors in order to avoid the first surgery for cartilage biopsy and subsequent chondrocyte cell cultivation. Authors have recognized that nucleated cells found in bone marrow are a useful source of cells for restoration of damaged tissue[8,9]; furthermore, using MSC and Platelet Rich Plasma (PRP), it is possible to repair cartilage in a one-step procedure[10].

MSC have a high proliferation and multi-lineage differentiation potential, into adipogenic, osteogenic and chondrogenic cells[11].

Many authors have shown in animal and laboratory studies the use of mesenchymal stem cells with chondrogenic potential but only few clinical studies have been done[10,11,12,13,14,15].

Once MSC are cultured in the appropriate microenvironment, they can differentiate to chondrocytes and form cartilage; onset of chondrogenesis requires a chemically defined serum free medium supplemented with dexamethasone, ascorbic acid and growth factors such as TGF-B[8].

The micromass culture or pellet culture system is generally considered a good in vitro model of chondrogenesis; Johnstone et al.[11] cultured MSC as pellets at the bottom of a tube for 2 weeks in a specific serum free cocktail medium; under these conditions cells organize a cartilaginous matrix by secreting proteoglycans and type II collagen and cells appear as real chondrocytes embedded in their own matrix lacunae.

Nixon et al.[10] showed early-enhanced chondrogenesis in cartilage defects in an equine model, he concluded that MSC arthroscopic implantation in horses improved cartilage healing response.

Research are currently exploring the possibility of implanting stem cells in the laboratory to differentiate into chondrocytes and which can then be utilized with a synthetic scaffold[12,13] or scaffold free[14] for implantation.

Ochi et al.[15] observed that in a rat model the injection of cultured MSC combined with bone marrow stimulation can accelerate the regeneration of articular cartilage; they noted that this cell therapy was a less invasive treatment for cartilage injury. In their other animal study[16] they introduced a MSC delivery system with the help of an electromagnetic field, enhancing the proliferation of cartilage inside the chondral defect after intra-articular injection, decreasing ectopic cartilage formation. Fortier et al.[17] concluded, in their animal studies that development of patient-side configuration techniques for intra-operative stem cell isolation and purification for immediate grafting have significant advantages in time savings and immediate application of an autogenous cell for cartilage repair.

Wakitani et al.[18] used autologous culture of expanded bone marrow for repair of cartilage defects in osteoarthritic knees; they chose 24 knees of 24 patients with knee OA who underwent a high tibial osteotomy; patients were divided into cell transplanted group and cell free group. After 16 months follow-up, they concluded that MSC were capable of regenerating a repair tissue for large chondral defects.

Our institution also use bone marrow concentrated (BMC) for MSC in treating chondral defects: our technique consists of harvesting 40-60 mL of bone marrow aspirate from the iliac crest (Fig 1) with aspiration kit and a centrifugations system (Harvest SmartPReP®2 System - Harvest Technologies corp., Plymouth, USA, Extracell-Regen Lab, Mollens, CH) following the method recommended by the manufacturer in order to have BMC and from these we will be able to increase concentration of BMC four to six times the baseline value.

Using Batroxobin enzyme (Plateltex®act-Plateltex S.R.O. Bratislava, SK)[19] we activate the bone marrow concentrate and produce a sticky clot material that we paste it into the defect; (Fig 2-3) finally we use to cover the treated defect with a collagenic membrane, (ChondroGide® Geistlich, Wolhusen, CH) (Fig 4).

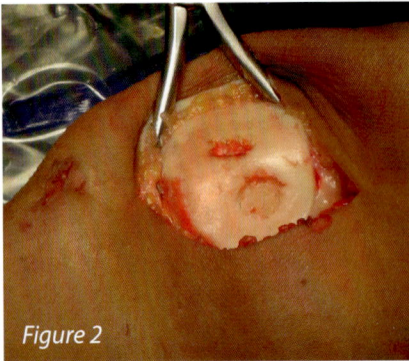

Figure 2

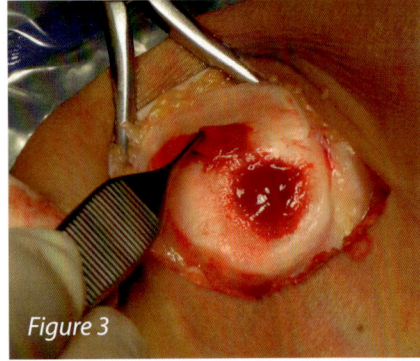

Figure 3

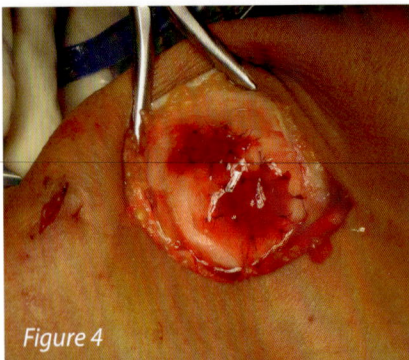

Figure 4

Figure 2: Patellar lesions.

Figure 3: Pasting MSC:s and membrane.

Figure 4: Final view after membrane suture.

Preliminary data from our institution and other Italian authors on MSC implantation with a one-step procedure seem to be promising, showing good clinical outcomes at early follow up. Giannini et al.[20] presented their one step surgery procedure using MSC and scaffold. 20 patients with a mean age of 26 years of age with chondral lesions were treated. Patients were evaluated using clinical scores and MRIs. They had a minimum of 6 months and maximum 24 months follow up. IKDC subjective and objective scores showed significant improvement from pre-op to final follow up. MRI evaluation showed progression of regeneration from pre-op to final follow-up.

We noted a trend towards improvement of the mean IKDC scores from 53.0 pre-op to 73.0 at final follow-up at two years. KOOS, Tegner and Lysholm showed similar trends[19].

Platelet Rich Plasma

Another interesting therapy is platelet-rich plasma. Platelet rich plasma contains 3-6 times platelets of normal blood and growth factors (platelet rich in growth factors or PRGF) in these platelets there is a high density of alpha granules, which contain proteins, furthermore, PRGF contains different growth factors, such as PDGF, IGF-1, TGF-B, EGF, bFGF, VEGF, and others[22]. They regulate key processes involved in tissue repair, including cell proliferation, chemotaxis, migration, cellular differentiation, and extracellular matrix synthesis .

Initially, it was used in transfusion medicine to treat hemorrhagic conditions secondary to thrombocytopenia, acute leukaemia or severe blood loss after surgery. Later this therapy enjoyed a great increase in popularity because of the versatility, biocompatibility and low-costs of this approach and has stimulated its therapeutic use in many medical field. Scientific research and technology has provided new insight in understanding the biological potential of platelet in wound and tissue healing process[23-26].

Cugat et al.[27] used PRGF to treat chondral defect in athletes and obtained good results, according to their experiences for other connective tissue repair, they showed that PRGF in physiological concentration is effective for the recovery of connective tissue furthermore local treatment is safe and does not alter the systemic concentrations of these proteins.

In Italy, Kon et al.[28] have studied a group of 30 patients with symptomatic degenerative disease of the knee joints treated with three PRP intra-articular injections weekly; the follow up at 6 months showed positive effects on the function and symptoms. Same authors recently presented their comparative study between Hyaluronic Acid (HA) and PRP injections: 91 patients with a mean age of 50.1 years with degenerative lesions and OA were followed up after injection of HA or PRP. Results were better in PRP group in clinical knee scores and pain score[29].

In our institution we use a Leukocyte rich -PRP according to Dohan et al classification[30] in treating early arthritis, ICRS grade 3-4. Among a group of 50 patients we followed-up 23 patients with a mean age of 44.3 years, 13 with previous knee surgeries. We collected pain visual analogue scale (VAS) and KOOS score at pre-treatment, 3 and 6 months post treatment, and the preliminary results are encouraging. There was a trend towards improvement in both scores[31].

Recently authors have proven synergistic effects of PRP combined with MSC, Nishimoto et al.[30] suggested that simultaneous concentration of PRP and bone marrow cells (BMC), acting as a sources of growth factors and "working cells", could play important roles in future regenerative medicine. Drengk et al.[33] exhibited in their study that a combination of Platelet rich plasma and MSC 14 fold increase in cell proliferation and would form a bioactive composite suited for healing of cartilage defects in vivo. These results were also evident in an in vivo study done by Milano et al.[34] that showed a more effective cartilage repair after microfracture associated to hydrogel scaffold with PRP. Finally, several authors[35,36,37] have stated that growth factors could act like as a carrier to fix chondrocytes into cartilage defects and can be combined with mesenchymal stem cells.

Preliminary data are encouraging; however, further studies on clinical efficacy will clarify if simultaneous use of PRP and MSC could represent a real solution for regenerative medicine in cartilage repair. These studies show less morbidities and complications inherent to cartilage surgical techniques by lessening surgical procedures translating to lower cost for the patient. However medium term prospective randomized studies are suggested to confirm these preliminary results.

Gene therapy

Therapeutic gene transfer into articular cartilage is a potential means to stimulate reparative activities in tissue lesions. The spontaneous repair in such articular cartilage defects shares interesting similarities with the embryonic chondrogenesis. Initially, the defect is filled with mesenchymal cells arising from the bone marrow. These cells proliferate and differentiate into chondrocytes, which deposit a matrix rich in types I and II collagen. After some months, the defect has been filled with a repair tissue that resembles articular cartilage. However, for reasons that are unknown, this repair tissue degenerates over time and is not capable to withstand the forces of a joint. These chondrogenic processes are regulated by chondrogenic growth and transcription factors, among which Sox9, FGF-2, members of the BMP superfamily such as BMP-2, IGF-I and many others. This led to the idea of applying such factors to cartilage defects in order to modulate and further improve the chondrogenesis in these defects. However, application of growth factor proteins is hampered by their short pharmacological half-life. This has let to the application of gene transfer to achieve a localized delivery into the defect of therapeutic gene constructs. Among the most studied candidates, polypeptide growth factors have shown promise to enhance the structural quality of the repair tissue. We as many others have shown that over expression of growth and transcription factors via nonviral, recombinant adenoviral and recombinant adeno-associated virus (rAAV) vectors significantly improves the structure of the repair tissue in osteochondral defects in vivo. In the future, it will be important to enhance our understanding of the basic scientific aspects of chondrogenesis. This will, as a result, lead to a better knowledge of the molecular events that regulate the repair of articular cartilage defects and that are responsible for the degeneration of the repair tissue. Likewise, these studies will also result in the identification of novel molecular targets for articular cartilage repair. It will be important to identify and better characterize efficient and safe gene vectors. Cooperation of muscoloskeletal researchers in many specialized disciplines will successfully address these open questions.

Tissue engineering

The research on the identification or creation of the ideal material for engineering cartilage substitutes has been very prolific in the last decade. The use of polymers, both natural and synthetic, that undergo controllable bulk erosion or resorption have been largely investigated as they could represent a favourable solution for engineering cartilage tissues in vitro or in vivo. For example, polymers that degrade at a rate proportional to which cartilaginous extracellular matrix is being deposited into the intercellular spaces could be employed to generate cartilaginous tissue in situ. Several scaffolds, both natural and synthetic, have been tested in animal models for regenerating cartilage tissue. Whereas many favorable polymers are open lattice structures with large pores into which cartilage matrix is permitted to form, new synthetic hydrogels are also good candidate scaffolds for generating cartilage tissue.

Synthetic Polymers

Many early investigations for engineering cartilage from synthetic polymers focused on the use of polyesters of poly(α-hydroxy esters)[38]. Biodegradable polyesters such as poly(L-lactic acid) (PLLA), poly(glycolic) acid (PGA), and the copolymer poly(DL-lactic-coglycolic acid) (PLGA), possess many desired properties to support cell transplantation.

Biological Scaffolds

Collagen is the prevalent structural biomolecule in the extracellular matrix of cartilage, making it a logical choice for composing a tissue engineering scaffold. Collagen sponges have many desirable properties as a biological scaffold for cartilage, including porosity, biodegradability, and biocompatibility. Open lattice collagen scaffolds, some of which also include glycosaminoglycans, have been synthesized and used for generating new cartilage matrix. Scaffolds made from a single collagen type or composites of two or more types have been employed. Following the list of the potential biological scaffolds for cartilage repair, hyaluronan could play an important role. It is one of the major constituents of undifferentiated mesenchyme in the developing embryo as well as in the cartilage extracellular matrix. Hyaluronan has been shown to support proliferation of mesenchymal progenitor cells and differentiation into chondrocytes. Additionally, in cartilage it is believed to play a significant role in physical microenvironment affecting chondrocyte function.

Hydrogel Scaffolds

The inability to deliver chondrocytes through minimally invasive techniques when using fibrous or open lattice-type polymers stimulated investigations into other types of polymer carriers such as hydrogels, which are gelatinous colloids that when maintained under controlled conditions exhibit three-dimensional stability. As the polymer gels, there is usually sufficient opportunity to mold and shape the final three-dimensional configuration of the gel. Additionally, by existing in a liquid phase, these polymers have the potential for injectable delivery. Hydrogels have proven to be extremely effective in providing a hospitable, three-dimensional support matrix for the immobilization of cells. By suspending chondrocytes in a highly porous aqueous matrix, they can maintain their differentiated function and are capable of producing large quantities of extracellular matrix macromolecules. Examples of hydrogels used to encapsulate chondrocytes include alginates and chitosan, hydrogen bonded block copolymers such as covalently crosslinked fibrin glue. Fibrin, which can be obtained from autologous blood products and is favorably biocompatible, can be formulated as an injectable vehicle with degradation controlled using agents like aprotinin that slow fibrinolysis. Various studies have focused on using chondrocytes in fibrin gel polymer as a hydrogel scaffold for engineering cartilage[39,40]. Elisseeff et al. have studied the potential of another interesting category of hydrogel having the characteristics of being photo-polimerizable, as for example poly(ethylene oxide) (PEO). They demonstrated that chondrocytes- PEO constructs could be injected subcutaneously, molded to the desired shape, and then polymerized transdermally with ultraviolet light[41]. Similar materials are recently approaching clinical use and can represent a valid alternative tool for cartilage repair in the future.

An important issue to be addressed for the future perspective for cartilage repair is the quality of the bonding and the integration of the newly formed tissue to the native tissue. Different studies were completed and all seem to demonstrate the importance to the presence of both cells and the newly synthesized matrix for achieving a stable healing[42,43]. It appears very interesting the extensive work done recently on generating composite tissues, in particular osteochondral substitutes[44,45]. Of particular interest are the studies of the production of multiple composite, which can be custom made based on the patients' defect[46]. This is possible thanks to the solid collaboration of experts from different disciplines, like chemistry, physics, biology, engineering, imaging, medicine and surgery, just for mentioning few. This possibly would lead to the generation of tissue engineered strategies for the repair of complex lesions involving cartilage, together with the subchondral bone and other structures, which is crucial for the wellbeing of the joint and therefore of the patient.

References

1. Hunter W: On the Structure and Diseases of Articulating Cartilage. PhilosTrans Rsoc Lond Biol Sci; 1743; 9: 277.
2. Ciombor DM, Aaron RK, Wang S, Simon B. Modification of osteoarthritis by pulsed electromagnetic field: A morphological study. Osteoarthritis Cartilage. 2003;11:455-462.
3. Massari L, Benazzo F, De Mattei M, Setti S, Fini M, CRES Study Group. Effects of electrical physical stimuli on articular cartilage. J Bone Joint Surg Am. 2007;89(suppl 3):152-161.
4. Peterson L, Minas T, Brittberg M et al. Treatment of Osteochondritis Dissecans of the Knee with

Autologous Chondrocyte Transplantation: Results at Two to Ten Years. J Bone Joint Surg Am. 2003; 85-A Suppl 3:17-24.

5. Mandelbaum, B. Next generation Cell Based Therapy. AANA 2007 Specialty Day San Diego, California. Final Program; 24-31. 2007.

6. Gobbi A, Kon E, Filardo G, Delcogliano M, Montaperto C, Boldrini L, Bathan L and Marcacci M. Patellofemoral Full-Thickness Chondral Defects Treated With Second Generation ACI: Results at 5 years Follow-up. Am J Sports Med. 2009 (In Press)

7. Marcacci M, Berruto M, Gobbi A, Kon E,. et al. Articular cartilage engineering with Hyalograft C: 3-year clinical results. Clin Orthop Relat Res.

8. Robey PG, Bianco P.The use of adult stem cells in rebuilding the human face. J Am Dent Assoc. 2006 Jul;137(7):961-72. Review.

9. Kobayashi T, Ochi M, Yanada S et al. A novel cell delivery system using magnetically labeled mesenchymal stem cells and an external magnetic device for clinical cartilage repair. Arthroscopy. 2008 Jan;24(1):69-76.

10. Nixon AJ, Wilke MM, Nydam DV. Enhanced early chondrogenesis in articular defects following arthroscopic mesenchymal stem cell implantation in an equine model. JOrthop Res. 2007 Jul;25(7):913-25.

11. Johnstone B, Hering TM, Caplan AI, et al. In vitro chondrogenesis of bone marrow-derived mesenchymal progenitor cells. Exp Cell Res. 1998 Jan 10;238(1):265-72.

12. Ando, W, Frank CB, Nakamura, D.A. et al. Comparisom of mesenchymal progenitor cellsderived from different pocrine tissues for lineage specific potential. ICRS Abstract Book: p75 Miami, USA. May, 2009.

13. Milkovic, N, Rubin, JP, Lin M. Chondrogenesis of Adipose-derived Stem Cells for Cartilage Repair. ICRS Abstract Book: p75 Miami, USA. May, 2009.

14. Ando W, Tateishi K, Katakai D, Hart DA, Higuchi C, Nakata K, Hashimoto J, Fujie H, Shino K, Yoshikawa H, Nakamura N. n vitro generation of a scaffold-free tissue-engineered construct (TEC) derived from human synovial mesenchymal stem cells: biological and mechanical properties and further chondrogenic potential. Tissue Eng Part A. 2008 Dec;14(12):2041-9.

15. Ochi M, Kanaya A, Nishimori M. Cell therapy for promotion of cartilage regeneration after drilling and ACL healing. 6TH Biennial ISAKOS Congress.

16. Ochi M, Adachi N, Nobuto H, Agung M, Kawamata S, Yanada S. Effects of CD44 antibody-or RGDS peptide--immobilized magnetic beads on cell proliferation and chondrogenesis of mesenchymal stem cells. J Biomed Mater Res A. 2006 Jun 15;77(4):773-84.

17. Fortier, LA, Nixon, AJ, Williams J, Cable, CS. W.V.O.C. Symposium Keystone CO, 2006

18. Wakitani S, Imoto K, Yamamoto T, et al. Human autologous culture expanded bone marrow mesenchymal cell transplantation for repair of cartilage defects in osteoarthritic knees. Osteoarthritis Cartilage. 2002 Mar;10(3):199-206.

19. Mazzucco L, Balbo V, Cattana E, Borzini P Platelet-rich plasma and platelet gel preparation using Plateltex. Vox Sang. 2008 Apr;94(3):202-8.

20. Gianini et al. One Step Surgery with Mesenchymal Stem Cells. Presented at Isokinetic 2009. Bologna, Italy.

21. Bathan, L, Bioldrini, L, and Gobbi, A. Mesenchymal Stem Cells Implantation For Full thickness Cartilage Lesions Treatment: Preliminary Report. Poster. ICRS Abstract Book: P249. Miami, USA. May, 2009.

22. Robert BD. The clinical and laboratory utility of platelet volume parameters. Aus J Med Sci. 1994; 14: 625- 41.

23. Fukumoto T, Sperling JW, Sanyal A, et al. Combined effects of insulin-like growth factor-1 and transforming growth factor-beta1 on periosteal mesenchymal cells during chondrogenesis in vitro. Osteoarthritis Cartilage. 2003 Jan;11(1):55-64.

24. Barry F, Boynton RE, Liu B, et al. Chondrogenic differentiation of mesenchymal stem cells from bone marrow: differentiation-dependent gene expression of matrix components. Exp Cell Res. 2001 Aug 15;268(2):189-200.

25. Stevens MM, Marini RP, Martin I, et al. FGF-2 enhances TGF-beta1-induced periosteal chondrogenesis. J Orthop Res. 2004 Sep;22(5):1114-9.

26. Anitua E, Sanchez M, orive G, Andia I. The potential impact of the preparation rich in growth factors (PRGF) in different medical fields. Biomaterials 2007;28:4551-4560.

27. Cugat R, Carrillo JM, Serra I, et al. Articular cartilage defects reconstruction by plasma rich growth factors. Basic science, clinical repair and reconstruction of articular cartilage defects: current status and prospects. TIMEO 801-807

28. Kon E. Utilisation of platelet-derived growth factors for the treatment of degenerative cartilage pathology. 7th World Congress of ICRS, Warsaw, October 2007

29. Kon, E, Buda, R et al. The Evolution of Arthritis: Growth Factors. Presented at Isokinetic 2009. Bologna, Italy.

30. Dohan Ehrenfest DM, Rasmusson L, Albrektssson T. Classification of platelet concentrates: from pure platelet-rich plasma (P-PRP) to leucocyte- and platelet-rich fibrin (L-PRF). Trends in Biotechnology, 2008; 27 (3): 158-167

31. Boldrini, L. Gobbi, A. Infiltrative Treatment With Autologous Platelet Rich Plasma In Early Osteoarthritis: Our Experience. Presented at Isokinetic 2009. Bologna, Italy.

32. Nishimoto S, Oyama T, Matsuda K.Simultaneous concentration of platelets and marrow cells: a simple and useful technique to obtain source cells and growth factors for regenerative medicine. Wound Repair Regen. 2007 Jan-Feb;15(1):156-62

33. Drengk A, Zapf A, Sturmer E, Sturmer K, Frosch K, Influence of Platelet – Rich Plasma on Chondrogenic Differentiation and Proliferation of Chondrocytes and Mesenchymal Stem Cells. Cells Tissues and Organs 2008 :10.1159.

34. Milano G, Zarelli D et al. Does Platelet Rich Plasma Injection enhance Cartilage Healing After Microfractures? An Animal Study. Poster no. 536. 54th Annual Meeting of the Orthopaedic Research Society.

35. Espregueira-Mendes, J. Influence of Platelet Rich Plasma on Chondrogenic Differentiation and proliferation of chondrocytes.

36. Wu W, Chen F, Liu Y, Ma Q, Mao T. Autologous Injectable Tissue-Engineered Cartilage by Using Platelet-Rich Plasma: Experimental Study in a Rabbit Model. Journal of Oral and Maxillofacial Surgery, 2007 65 1951-1957.

37. Graziani F, Ivanovski S, Cei S, Ducci F, Tonetti M, Gabriele M. The in vitro effect of different PRP concentrations on osteoblasts and fibroblasts. Clin Oral Implants Res. 2006 Apr;17(2):212-9.

38. Langer R, Vacanti JP. Tissue Engineering. Science 260: 920-926, 1993

39. Peretti GM, Randolph MA, Villa MT, Buragas MS, Yaremchuk MJ. Cell/Based Tissue Engineered Allogeneic Implant for Cartilage Repair. Tissue Eng 6(5): 567-576, 2000

40. Peretti GM, Randolph MA, Zaporojan V, Bonassar LJ, Xu JW, Fellers J, Yaremchuk MJ. A biomechanical analysis of an engineered cell-scaffold implant for cartilage repair. Ann Plast Surg 46(5);533-37, 2001

41. Elisseeff J, Anseth K, Sims D, McIntosh W, Randolph M, Yaremchuk M, Langer R. Transdermal photopolymerization of poly(ethylene oxide)-based injectable hydrogels for tissue-engineered cartilage. Plast Reconstr Surg 104(4):1014-1022, 1999

42. Peretti GM, Randolph MA, CarusoEM, Rossetti F and Zaleske DJ. Bonding of cartilaginous matrices with cultured chondrocytes: an experimental model. J Orthop Res16(1):89-95, 1998

43. Peretti GM, Zaporojan V, Spangenberg KM, Randolph MA, Fellers J, Bonassar LJ. Cell-based bonding of articular cartilage: an extended study. J Biomed Mater Res, 1;64A(3):517-24, 2003

44. Mano JF, Reis RL. Osteochondral defects: present situation and tissue engineering approaches. J Tissue Eng Regen Med. 2007 Jul-Aug;1(4):261-73

45. Scotti C., Buragas M.S., Mangiavini L., Sosio C., Di Giancamillo A., Domeneghini C., Fraschini G., Peretti G.M. A tissue engineered osteochondral plug: an in vitro morphological evaluation. Knee Surg Sports Traumatol Arthrosc 2007 Nov;15(11):1363-9

46. Grayson, WL et al. Trends in Biotecnology 2008; vol 26(4)